GRID APPROACHES FOR MANAGERIAL LEADERSHIP IN NURSING

GRID APPROACHES FOR MANAGERIAL LEADERSHIP IN NURSING

ROBERT R. BLAKE, Ph.D.

JANE SRYGLEY MOUTON, Ph.D.

MILDRED TAPPER, Ph.D.

The C. V. Mosby Company

ST. LOUIS • TORONTO • LONDON   1981

The C. V. Mosby Company
11830 Westline Industrial Drive, St. Louis, Missouri 63141

Library of Congress Cataloging in Publication Data

Blake, Robert Rogers, 1918-
  Grid approaches for managerial leadership in
nursing.

  Bibliography: p.
  Includes index.
    1. Nursing service administration. I. Mouton,
Jane Srygley, joint author. II. Tapper, Mildred,
1925-   joint author. III. Title. [DNLM:
1. Nursing, Supervisory. WY105 B636g]
RT89.B52   610.73′068   80-21583
ISBN 0-8016-0696-9

AC/M/M 9 8 7 6 5 4 3 2 1   05/B/599

PREFACE

This book is for those concerned with nursing administration: students at all levels interested in nursing leadership and management, the director of nursing, the head nurse, the charge nurse, the supervisor, and the staff nurse who is the one most directly responsible for primary patient care. All of these either administer nursing practices or receive administration from others. It is written to aid those who study and practice nursing administration to see the options available for achieving excellence in patient care with and through those who are more directly related to the patient than the administrator herself.

Her responsibility is exercised with and through those intermediate between herself and the patient. That is what nursing administration is all about—mobilizing the resources that staff nurses and others are capable of contributing toward the end of excellence in patient care.

For purposes of illustration, the head nurse is the administrative professional who is concentrated upon from the standpoint of the examples provided in this book. The character, if not the content, of administration is the same, however, regardless of who is supervising whom. Supervision is the issue of importance, and the human factor is the critical aspect of it.

The feminine gender is used throughout the book, although we recognize that many men are engaged in or entering the nursing profession.

This book provides the reader a clear way of discriminating between strong, sound supervision and supervision that is less adequate. *Grid Approaches for Managerial Leadership in Nursing* is a theoretical framework for seeing these distinctions in specific, concrete ways. Its value is in aiding the nurse to consider alternative ways of supervision, or "measuring" herself in the context of these alternatives and determining her own characteristic style. Then she can plot a course of change so that less effective supervisory practices can be replaced by others that aid her to avoid past difficulties and gain future benefits.

The collaboration that has produced this book is an interesting and mutually rewarding one. Internationally known as the developers of Grid concepts, Drs. Robert Blake and Jane Mouton have worked together for many years and have used the Grid to investigate sound and unsound practices in a number of very basic human relationships, such as between supervisor and subordinate in industry or government, salesman and customer, husband and wife, and so on.* The first edition of *The New Managerial Grid* has become a classic management text, with the Grid having been used for two decades as the basic reference for development programs for industrial, service, and research companies and government agencies. The third author, Dr. Mildred Tapper, brings years of direct experience in nursing and as head nurse in several hospitals. At Massachusetts General Hospital she initiated a program to prepare head nurses for this position. Her contribution is reinforced by having taught at Boston University School of Nursing. She is currently associate professor at The University of Texas in Austin, School of Nursing.

Ms. Artie Stockton facilitated the project in many ways: organizing the writing activities, editing, and supervising the preparation of the manuscript.

Our objective has been to provide a conceptual framework within which the problems of managerial leadership in nursing can clearly be seen and in this way to contribute to the administration of primary patient care.

Robert R. Blake
Jane Srygley Mouton
Mildred Tapper

---

*Grid® is a registered trademark of Scientific Methods, Inc., P.O. Box 195, Austin, Texas 78767.

CONTENTS

Chapter 1

THE NURSE GRID

The nurse is a key professional in hospital management. Her supervision converts policies and prescriptions into daily practices that impact on the patient's experience in the hospital.

The nursing administrator plans, schedules, organizes, directs, and performs other administrative functions.[1] She gets her results, her production, by working with and through other nurses, becoming active in primary patient care only under unique circumstances. The staff members are the ones who actually get the job done. The nursing administrator may or may not see staff members as people who have positive and negative feelings and emotions, who can think constructively about solving problems, and who may be well motivated to do the best work possible in making the hospital function. Therefore the focus of this book is on the nurse who provides managerial leadership; in this case, the head nurse, and those with whom she works. The Grid is used to investigate how she leads in everyday work.

The head nurse as an administrator has two major concerns. The first is for production or results: providing all those activities essential for patient care. This concern means many things. One is seeing to it that procedures are carried out—that staff members take blood pressure and temperatures, give medications as prescribed, start and maintain IV's, and take whatever actions are okayed under standing orders. It also means overseeing the bathing of patients, the changing of beds, and the housekeeping of patient quarters and other unit facilities. It mean conveying to the patient or others information necessary for care after discharge. It means filing incident reports as well as taking necessary action to rectify any problems being encountered. Since the head nurse is in an administrative capacity, it also means orienting new employees, scheduling training, administering procedures and policies, and so on. All of these duties come together in the form of *concern for hospital services*. These are services that support a patient while in the hospital. The shorthand for this is *concern for production*.

The second concern is for the hospital personnel as persons. This *concern for other persons* is evident in the way information is given, the quality of listening for feedback, the manner in which mistakes are dealt with, the quality of consideration shown when special needs arise, and in a host of other ways. These are all the individuals who are responsible for delivering the services just described.

THE GRID

Concern for production and concern for staff members as persons are expressed in vastly different ways, depending on the specific manner in which these two concerns mesh. High concern for production coupled with low concern for staff, or a high concern for staff coupled with a low concern for production, are significantly different ways of supervising.[2] These are both different than the kind of high concern for a staff member that is joined with an equally high concern for productivity.

These two concerns may come together in many combinations, and the interactions between them determine the foundation of a nurse's supervisory

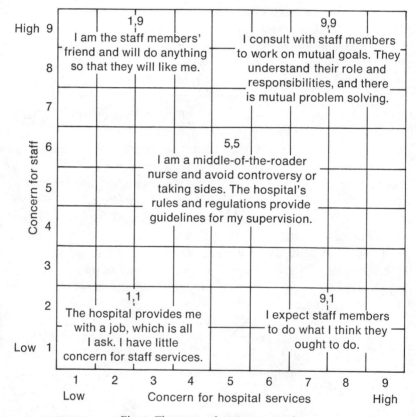

Fig. 1. The nurse administrator Grid.

style.[3] Fig. 1 shows the range of possible couplings. The horizontal axis indicates concern for production of hospital services. The vertical axis indicates concern for staff members as people. Each is a nine-point scale, with 1 representing a minimum concern, 5 symbolizing an intermediate degree of concern, and 9 representing maximum concern. There are 81 possible combinations of these concerns represented on the Grid. Next to 9,1 are 8,2 and 7,3. Near to 1,9 are 2,8 and 3,7. Then there are 3,3, 4,4, 6,6, 7,7 on the diagonal between 1,1 and 9,9 and so on.

Each of these 81 positions on the Grid is a theory of how the head nurse thinks about the relationship between the care given patients and the staff responsible for giving the care. The various theories on the Grid can aid a nursing administrator to understand her own behavior as well as the reactions of the staff nurses and others she supervises. Theory is a valuable tool for helping a nurse see the assumptions on which her behavior is based.[4] With a sound understanding of her own behavior, the administrative nurse is then in a position to strive toward excellence in the performance of her duties and in helping others do their best.

Going around the Grid

The main emphasis is to be placed on the theories in the corners and in the middle of the Grid, as shown in Fig. 1. These are the most distinctive theories. They are the ones seen most often in day-by-day supervision. No doubt, as you consider each Grid style, an administrative nurse you know will come into your mind as fitting that particular style. Later on you will have an opportunity to diagnose your own style.

In the lower right corner is the style of a 9,1-oriented administrative nurse. Here high concern for delivering hospital services, 9, is coupled with little or no concern for staff as individual persons with thoughts and feelings, or 1. Pressure for results is applied on a "do as I say" basis.

In the upper left corner of the Grid is the 1,9-oriented theory. A minimum concern for administering hospital services is joined with a maximum concern for staff nurses and other hospital personnel. This nurse is concerned first with developing friendly relations with staff. She "knows" that when she offers them her warmth and approval they will carry out their nursing duties in a professional manner, without having to be told much of anything. She believes that staff members blossom when warm, supportive, nondirective and nonjudgmental supervision is provided.

In the lower left corner is the 1,1-oriented strategy of supervision. Here, concern for services and concern for the staff are both at a low ebb. You may think it odd that a nursing administrator could have almost no concern for either providing needed services or for those she supervises. She has not physically quit, but she has mentally left the health care organization. This nurse goes through the motions of being part of the organization but does not really contribute to it. Such nurses exist, but this strategy is easy to overlook, partly because they get by on a "see no evil, hear no evil, speak no evil" basis.

In the center is the 5,5-oriented Grid style of hospital supervision. This is the "middle of the road" strategy based on maintaining an intermediate amount of both concerns. The nurse supervising in this way wants her staff to maintain a steady pace that is acceptable to all. She relies on policy manuals and procedural guidelines in making decisions so that she does not have to take sides.

The upper right corner is the 9,9-oriented supervisory position. This couples high concern for delivery of hospital services with a high concern for personnel as individuals. The nurse with this orientation leads by gaining the involvement, participation, and commitment of staff nurses and others to achieve mutually shared goals. Staff members working together in a 9,9 manner know that they have a common stake in the outcome of their endeavors through better health care delivery carried out in a personally rewarding and satisfying way.

These Grid positions are described in more detail in subsequent chapters. Each demonstrates a different style of supervision employed on a day-by-day basis. Once a supervisor understands these theories of hospital supervision, then she will be able to see their consequences for good or poor care of patients. In addition, maternalism and other combinations of basic Grid styles are also dealt with later in the book.

Dominant and backup styles

A person's Grid style is quite consistent over a range of situations, but it is also true that individuals shift from one Grid style to another, sometimes even on a moment-by-moment basis. How can we shift and change if most of us have one dominant set of Grid assumptions? The answer is that, not only do most people have a dominant Grid style, but each of us also has a backup style; sometimes even a third, fourth, and fifth. A person's backup style becomes evident when it is difficult or impossible to apply the dominant or most characteristic Grid style. It is the style reverted to when a person is under pressure, tension, or strain, frustrated, or in situations of conflict that cannot be solved in his or her characteristic way.

Relationships between dominant and backup styles sometimes can be seen quite easily. How superiors deal with subordinates is a good basis for looking at this. First logic and reason are tried, reinforced with emotional acceptance in a

9,9 way. Failing to get a satisfactory response from subordinates, the supervisor uses a 5,5 approach, resulting in a compromise, so that both superior and subordinates feel at least partially satisfied. When this does not work, the superior gets tough and possibly adds a touch of ridicule, both 9,1 ways of trying to get the subordinates' attention. Then, since resentment and rejection have been created, she switches over to warmth and kindness and hopes that a 1,9 attitude will bring them around. Finally, still unable to elicit cooperation, she either returns to a 9,1 strategy of threats and punishments or throws up her hands in a 1,1 way and says, "Who cares?" Of course, this is only one sequence introduced to show dominant to backup. Another sequence may begin with a 9,1 or 1,1 or 1,9 or 5,5 approach.

There appear to be few, if any, strong natural or preferred links between any one Grid style as dominant and any other as backup. This great array of dominant-backup combinations contributes to making each person a unique individual. The point is that Grid styles are not fixed.

ASSUMPTIONS AND GRID POSITIONS

Each of the Grid theories is based on a different set of basic assumptions under which people engaged in work deal with one another.[5] An assumption is what one takes for granted as being true or reliable. People do not often question their basic assumptions. So if you, as a nurse administrator, were to interact with someone without making assumptions, you would have no strategy of supervision at all. Your behavior would be directionless.

Even so, it is not enough just to have a set of assumptions. Faulty assumptions lead to ineffective supervision. Getting to know your assumptions is a way of checking out your strategies and examining alternative assumptions that might make you more effective.

When a nursing administrator, acting under a given set of assumptions, understands them, Grid knowledge can aid her to predict what the impact of her behavior will be on staff members, colleagues, patients, and others. Therefore, learning the Grid framework helps her understand what kinds of actions are likely to lead to what kinds of results. It can help her examine alternative assumptions and how these function under different Grid strategies. Once a nurse identifies what reduces her effectiveness as a leader, she is progressing toward making a change in the direction of greater effectiveness. Once she can see how much more effective she can be by doing something different, her progress toward effectiveness can accelerate. The emphasis in this book is on introspection and self-appraisal. The ultimate primary interest is to help the patient receive the best care through nurses providing patient services in the soundest possible way.

There are basic forces at work that determine the strategies you as a nursing administrator employ. These are:

1. Immediate situations—that is, emergencies, time pressures, resistance from hospital personnel, high patient census.
2. Your requirements, real or imagined, of the agency, such as policies and procedures, past and present.
3. Your own Grid style.

Of all these forces, the one you can readily do something about is your own behavior. The next one you may be able to influence is the staff. The assumptions the staff reveals in dealing with you as the nurse can also be identified to aid you in understanding them.

THE PLAN OF THE BOOK

The nursing administrator exists in a world of great complexity. The manner in which she manages her relations with her superiors, colleagues, and subordinates all reflect her basic and backup Grid style.

Each style of supervision—9,1, 1,9, 1,1, 5,5, and 9,9—will be discussed in a chapter. These leadership styles influence behavior on the job in many ways. For the purpose of this book, eight different activities will be described to show how a nurse administrator operates within any given Grid style. These activities include:

1. Nurse in the middle.
2. Planning and scheduling.
3. Execution.
4. Follow-up.
5. Communication.
6. Conflict.
7. Development.
8. Introduction of change.

Before examining Grid styles in detail you will see that Chapter 2 provides an opportunity for you to evaluate your own Grid style. By completing the questions *before* you know more about the Grid you can get a snapshot of your own Grid style.

Chapter 2

SEEING YOURSELF IN THE NURSING ADMINISTRATOR GRID MIRROR

Before getting into a description of the circumstances involved in supervising the staff in a hospital agency, let us take a quick glance at you. This can help you to look beneath the surface and see yourself as a person with a dominant Grid style.

GRID ELEMENTS

Six elements describe qualities of personal behavior through which you can see your own Grid assumptions.[6] These elements are decisions, convictions, conflict, temper, humor, and energetic enthusiasm.

Five different sentences are provided under each element. Consider each sentence as a possible description of yourself in relation to that element. Place a 5 beside the sentence you think is most like yourself—the *actual* you, not the ideal you. Be as honest as you can.

Place a 4 beside the sentence you think is next most like yourself. Continue ranking the other sentences with 3 for the third, 2 for the fourth, and 1 for the fifth place, which is that sentence *least* characteristic of you. There can be no ties.

Reaching a decision is fundamental to any action. The point at which a person is committed to one course of action or another indicates the degree of certainty in making that choice. A head nurse who can look at a situation, read the facts, and reach a decision is seen as confident in her ability to solve problems. This confidence promotes confidence in others. One who is wishy-washy increases uncertainty in others regarding her own soundness.

Element 1: Decisions

_____ A1.   I accept the decisions of others with indifference.
_____ B1.   I support decisions that promote good relations.
_____ C1.   I search for workable, even though not perfect, decisions.
_____ D1.   I expect decisions I make to be treated as final.
_____ E1.   I place high value on getting sound, creative decisions that result in understanding and agreement.

In a society in which people are expected to think for themselves, the most highly respected are those who have sound convictions and hold to them. When a person has clear convictions, life has a sense of purpose, character, and direction. Individuals without convictions appear to others as weak, insecure, uncertain, anxious, or just plain indifferent to real issues.

Element 2: Convictions

_____ A2.   I avoid taking sides by not revealing opinions, attitudes, and ideas.
_____ B2.   I embrace opinions, attitudes, and ideas of others rather than push my own.
_____ C2.   When others hold ideas, opinions, or attitudes different from my own, I try to meet them halfway.
_____ D2.   I stand up for my ideas, opinions, and attitudes, even though it sometimes results in stepping on toes.
_____ E2.   I listen for and seek out ideas, opinions, and attitudes different from my own. I have clear convictions but respond to ideas sounder than my own by changing my mind.

Disagreement and conflict are inevitable in a culture in which people have different points of view and readily express them. Conflict can be either disruptive and destructive or creative and constructive, depending upon how it is met and handled. A person who can face conflict with another and resolve it to mutual understanding evokes respect and admiration. Inability to cope with conflict constructively and creatively leads to disrespect or oftentimes to increased hostility and antagonism. One makes a relationship; the other breaks it.

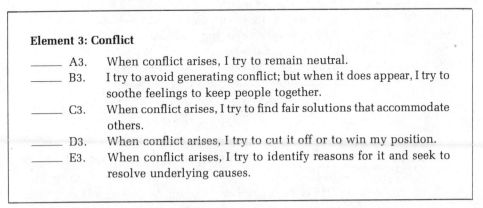

Element 3: Conflict

_____ A3. When conflict arises, I try to remain neutral.

_____ B3. I try to avoid generating conflict; but when it does appear, I try to soothe feelings to keep people together.

_____ C3. When conflict arises, I try to find fair solutions that accommodate others.

_____ D3. When conflict arises, I try to cut it off or to win my position.

_____ E3. When conflict arises, I try to identify reasons for it and seek to resolve underlying causes.

Temper is an emotional reaction to stress, tension, and strain. Loss of temper means that reason has been abandoned and violent, negative emotions have taken over. The loss of temper also has contagious effects. Its destructive qualities can spread like wildfire. But when an individual maintains a steady head and a strong hand, others have confidence that this person relies on reason and they respect her leadership. Persons who withhold their involvement and concern to keep from being stirred up are suspect. They may even be seen as not understanding the urgency of the problem.

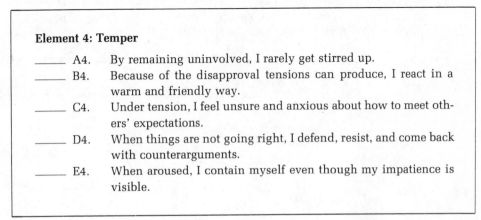

Element 4: Temper

_____ A4. By remaining uninvolved, I rarely get stirred up.

_____ B4. Because of the disapproval tensions can produce, I react in a warm and friendly way.

_____ C4. Under tension, I feel unsure and anxious about how to meet others' expectations.

_____ D4. When things are not going right, I defend, resist, and come back with counterarguments.

_____ E4. When aroused, I contain myself even though my impatience is visible.

Humor brings perspective to situations of strain and impasse, as well as gives richness to contradictory events. A person with sound humor contributes to the enjoyment of others. A person who is humorless is seen as lifeless and having no fun. One brings people toward her; the other lets them walk away.

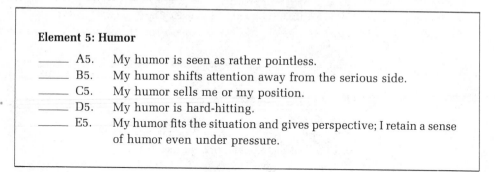

Element 5: Humor

_____ A5.   My humor is seen as rather pointless.

_____ B5.   My humor shifts attention away from the serious side.

_____ C5.   My humor sells me or my position.

_____ D5.   My humor is hard-hitting.

_____ E5.   My humor fits the situation and gives perspective; I retain a sense of humor even under pressure.

Healthy people have the capacity for using their energy in positive and constructive ways. When they do, enthusiasm is contagious; others catch it. It produces a "Can do!" spirit of optimism and progress. When people do not have enthusiasm, life is drab and conversation is dull and boring. Then pessimism creeps in, hopelessness appears, and a sense of "Why try?" results.

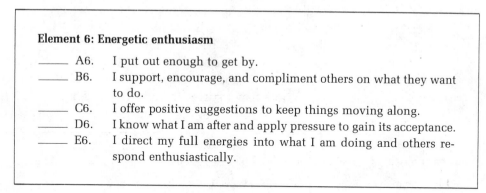

Element 6: Energetic enthusiasm

_____ A6.   I put out enough to get by.

_____ B6.   I support, encourage, and compliment others on what they want to do.

_____ C6.   I offer positive suggestions to keep things moving along.

_____ D6.   I know what I am after and apply pressure to gain its acceptance.

_____ E6.   I direct my full energies into what I am doing and others respond enthusiastically.

At this point there are two questions you might be asking. One is, "Are all the elements equally important in making up a nurse's Grid style?" The other is, "Are there no other equally important elements?"

The answer to the first question is, "no." They are not of equal importance. The *conflict* element appears to be the most central. You will see how important conflict is in the hospital situation when you often must deal with objections, resistance, and complaints, or with staff members who say one thing and do another. When you know a person's reaction to conflict, you tend to find that other elements fall in place around that reaction. That is why it is most important.

Are there other elements that make up a person's character? Yes, of course. Take for example such matters as personal integrity and thoroughness in pursuing knowledge, both about the immediate problem itself and about the staff member's approach to life. In later chapters, it will be seen that these aspects of a person's basic Grid style also are of significance.

The six elements are fundamental for clear understanding of the assumptions that head nurses make. They are also foundation stones for understanding the personal characteristics of a staff member. As you read, place yourself, as a nurse if you are now employed, in as many of these situations being illustrated as you possibly can. Imagine the situation or think what your reactions might be if you were a nurse in training. Then we will return to these rankings after you have read the next several chapters. Chapter 9 helps you to interpret the rankings you have just completed and to evaluate their implications for your supervisory effectiveness.

Chapter 3

THE 9,1-ORIENTED NURSING ADMINISTRATOR

The 9,1-oriented nursing administrator strives to be a powerful person. When she is, she feels secure, confident, on top. She submits to no one except when to do so is in the line of duty. If she is a director of nurses, the head nurse and staff nurses know very well who is boss. If she is a head nurse, she shows her power by being able to deliver what is asked of her by doctors and the director of nursing. Her power is also revealed in the way she controls and dominates the nurses on her staff. Whenever problems arise, she dictates the actions to be taken to prove herself capable of maintaining control. A 9,1-oriented nursing administrator places great importance on exercising her will-power, which she does almost inflexibly, determined to win by doing what is expected of her by her superiors, and by imposing her will on those who report to her regardless of opposition.

Sometimes a 9,1-oriented nurse does not get the results anticipated, no matter how hard she tries, and she then feels a failure. Her greatest fear is to make a mistake or lose control by being successfully resisted by someone. When failure does occur, she blames it on others who have blocked her will: "Next time I'll be more in charge—never depend on anybody but myself."

In summary, to win by staying on top is what a 9,1-oriented nurse strives for most; losing out and coming out on the bottom is what she seeks most to avoid.

Whatever is expected from above is what the nursing administrator seeks to get, and she expects compliance from others. After all, authority is to be respected. She gives no less loyalty to her superiors than she expects from her staff. So she acts under instruction on a "let the chips fall where they may" basis. Therefore she would not feel compelled to ask for a review of a decision because of the possible tension it might generate from those below, as this is not her way of managing. Another way of saying it is, when faced with a conflict of interest, the nursing administrator, under a 9,1 orientation, identifies with the position of greatest authority and power at whatever expense to her staff members or others.

Consider the nurse's station, for example. That is a 9,1-oriented head nurse's command post. Here she sets up the boundary lines and establishes her territory. Each staff nurse knows what space she can and cannot use, and no one had better be caught sitting in the head nurse's chair when she is around.

Now we can study these motivations as revealed in her approach to supervision of her own staff.

Production is all important. That is what she is employed to get and in the most efficient and economical way possible. It is what she measures herself against, certainly the key factor in promotion. Therefore, the 9,1-oriented nurse makes every effort to concentrate on doing her job—keeping the doctors from yelling or complaining, eliminating mistakes, staying on schedule, administering policy and procedures—and penalizing those who fail to do their part. After all, it is her crew, her ship.

NURSE IN THE MIDDLE

The nursing administrator—whether she is a director of nursing, a head nurse, or a charge nurse—is always caught between two human levels. The director of nurses may find herself caught between the hospital administrator's dictates and the doctors' wishes. She may find herself settling disputes between a department head and the ICU nurses.

The same is true of a head nurse.[7] As an administrator of a unit, she is responsible to the director of nurses. The administrator in charge of the hospital also refers changes to her. She is in between all the doctors, all the departments, the patients' families and friends, and is expected to be a staff representative. The staff nurse functions between head nurse and doctor, doctor and family, doctor and patient. She must oftentimes be a combination of parent, spouse, confidante, counselor, etc., fitting these in among administrative and medical duties that are required to support her patient care.

Her in-the-middle stance may be anything but nonpartisan because she takes the doctor's position almost blindly. Department heads and staff nurses come and go, but doctors are more or less permanent fixtures. They are her true allies.

The 9,1-oriented nursing administrator does not tolerate short circuiting of official channels. Since she is in the middle—either between the nurses and administration, between the doctors and administration, between the nurses and the doctors, between patients and doctors—the person who goes over her head either to the doctor regarding some patient problem or to administration about a policy or procedure is committing a cardinal sin. The nurse sees this as weakening her capacity to control what is going on; thus, questioning her authority is unacceptable. She does not feel that it is her responsibility to explain the policies and procedures that come down from administration. Subordinates who are offered explanations, she thinks, may retaliate by questioning policy, and there is little time to explain, much less justify, policies and procedures that have already been decided.

Many times, as the person in the middle, the nurse is told about changes that she knows will have a bad effect on staff members under her. Caught between what she is told to do from above and what she knows will cause trouble, frustration, anxiety, or insecurity, she can run into problems in her enforcement efforts.

Lana Johnson is a 9,1-oriented director of nurses at Middle City Hospital. She reacts in a hostile manner to Jean, a head nurse who is tense and frustrated from overtime work.

It is two o'clock Saturday afternoon when the victims of the explosion at a downtown building begin to arrive in the emergency room. When Lana arrives at the hospital, the doctors are triaging the patients as quickly as they can, but they need help badly. She begins to telephone off-duty doctors and nurses, but because it is the weekend, several staff nurses cannot be reached. Pressure continues to increase as doctors' tempers grow short and families and newspeople want to know what is going on.

At seven o'clock in the evening Lana is still coordinating the problem of getting extra beds, trying to contact replacement doctors and nurses, getting additional blood, contacting victims' families, etc. She is hurrying from her office with instructions for one of the charge nurses when she is approached by Jean, a head nurse on one of the units.

"Lana, I've been here sixteen hours and I feel sick. When do you think I can get some relief? I haven't even been able to call my family. I really need a break."

Lana stares incredulously at Jean. "I don't have to explain to you, Jean, that we have an emergency. There is no time to think about yourself. The job has to be done."

This is a 9,1-oriented reaction of a nurse in the middle. She disregards Jean's approaching exhaustion because of the pressure above her to respond to what is needed, pressure from the doctors, and pressure from staff members. Lana makes no explanation as to why she cannot respond to Jean's request. At that particular time Jean is an indispensable pair of hands. Having been totally disregarded as a person, it is unlikely that Jean will return to work with high morale or to help willingly in the future.

ADMINISTRATIVE ASPECTS OF NURSING

The production requirements of patient care are revealed in the nursing administrator's attitudes toward planning and scheduling, execution, and follow-up.

Planning and scheduling

Planning is deciding what to do, how to do it, and who is to do it. We can consider how the 9,1-oriented nursing administrator deals with such matters in day-to-day activities.

The nursing administrator has a position of authority in the hierarchy and she knows it; no one doubts who calls the shots. The staff members are not expected to contribute ideas to the task since their job is to turn out results. In a nutshell, a 9,1-oriented supervisor thinks about herself in this way:

"As the nursing administrator, I make out the assignments, which indicate to the staff what to do, how, when, and with whom."

The job is defined in terms of operational requirements, since this makes it clear to those who must carry out the duties exactly what is to be done. This ensures that follow-up is easy to do since it is clear again whether the assignment has been completed precisely as indicated. There is little flexibility for changes, as this would throw the schedule off. Coffee times are assigned, as are lunch breaks, and no deviations are permitted. "If you miss your lunch break, tough." She makes out the individual plans to ensure that everyone is kept busy. At the worst, "Idle hands are a devil's workshop." At the best, "People who are not busy gossip and make themselves unhappy."

Sometimes unanticipated situations arise and schedules have to be rearranged or procedures replanned. The following example reveals how the 9,1-oriented head nurse, Katherine, steps in decisively to prevent chaos even though there are side effects in terms of subordinates' feelings of antagonism and resentment.

Katherine, head nurse at White General, calls all the staff nurses together about ten minutes before the 3 p.m. shift is due to come on. She comes directly to the point. "Rose just called in sick and won't be able to work the 3-11 shift. One of you will have to cover."

Barbara, one of the nurses, makes a face. "Why did she call so late? I have a date that I don't want to break."

"And I would never be able to get a sitter," interjects Susan, "and besides, I'm tired. Let the next shift cope with it. They surely won't be *that* busy."

Katherine's face flushes. "You know as well as I that three nurses cannot cover the 3-11 shift under normal circumstances, much less considering the possibility of emergencies. If you can't volunteer I'll just have to select someone. Sharon, you take it since you have tomorrow off."

"But I'm leaving town tonight," protests Sharon.

"You're not now," and with that Katherine turns briskly and leaves the group standing there.

Later, on answering Mrs. Jones' buzzer, Sharon swears under her breath as she jerks open the door to Mrs. Jones' room. Her resentment, though misdirected, soon comes through to Mrs. Jones. "What do you want now? I told you fifteen minutes ago it would be after four when the snack cart comes around." The ill-tempered behavior becomes tomorrow's complaint to Katherine, confirming to her that Sharon is a real problem.

In the example we see Katherine dealing with the unexpected problem in an efficient way. Someone is needed regardless of personal hardship. Katherine does not allow off-the-job commitments to stand in the way. What she fails to see is the damaging effect of her 9,1-oriented actions on the way in which Sharon deals with her patient after the meeting. Sharon's exasperation with Katherine cannot be expressed directly to her so she is abrupt and unfeeling in turn toward those in her care. When Katherine gets the complaint about Sharon from Mrs. Jones, she will see no connection between her own treatment of Sharon and Sharon's taking it out on Mrs. Jones.

Execution

Since the staff members are expected to carry out whatever they are told to do, directions are given in a clear-cut and detailed way, leaving little opportunity for a staff person to misunderstand what the nursing administrator wants done. There is even less opportunity to ask questions. Assignments are to be met; the staff is expected to do no more or no less than what they are told. "Yours is not to question why; yours is but to do or die."

The staff members are expected to carry out assignments in a straightforward way, do what they have been told, and take no liberties by imposing their own thoughts, guesswork, or interpretation of the best thing to do in situations they have not received instructions about.

"These are your assignments; if you have no questions, get on with them."

Because of these basic attitudes, when the nursing administrator outlines what is to be undertaken, and how, and when, and by what time it should be done, the staff nurse is expected to indicate that she is going to comply, and then to report when it is done.

One of the biggest problems in making assignments and ensuring that people work by them is from staff nurses who constantly place personal needs above the unit needs. In the following example, Sara, a 9,1-oriented head nurse, must deal with Sheila, the staff nurse who is seeking to shift her assignment after she has been given it far enough in advance to be able to plan her personal requirements around it.

About two months ago Sheila's daughter became engaged and she and her fiance have set the wedding date for this May, which is only three months away. Thursday a friend of hers is planning a tea and Sheila would like to have that day off to attend the tea and spend some time with her daughter.

Sheila looks at her watch as she folds the blood pressure cuff and puts it in the drawer. She has just checked her last patient and in ten minutes will be off for the day. There is just enough time to check with the head nurse, Sara, about Sheila switching shifts with someone else next Thursday.

Sheila sees Sara as soon as she rounds the corner to the nurse's station, and Sheila proceeds to ask for a shift of assignment on Thursday.

"Requests for time just make for problems. Rules on this floor say that changes should be made at least a month ahead of time. Rules are rules. Besides, I've got the time made out and I'm not changing it."

"But, Sara," protests Sheila, "Helen has already said she would switch with me."

"Sheila, if I do it for you, I'll have to do it for others—and you'll be asking again. Besides, you're getting the wedding day off."

This orientation clearly tells the staff that the unit comes first and that there are no "special cases." Special cases set precedents that bring an end to orderly carrying out of predetermined plans or indicate to the staff that the head nurse is playing favorites in letting some people upset the schedule to the detriment of others.

Follow-up

With clear-cut and specific assignments that are to be complied with, the 9,1-oriented nursing administrator views her follow-up responsibilities as maintaining surveillance over the operations as they unfold in order to catch problems that occur.

"I keep in close touch with what's going on to ensure that everyone is following my instructions down to the last detail. I can't afford to let anything slip."

She knows, however, that things never go according to plan, people being what they are, and therefore it is up to her to keep things on track. In the following example, Grace, head nurse, keeps an eye on Joan, who has a habit of falling behind.

Joan, a staff nurse, goes in to give Mrs. Smith her bath. Joan is running behind schedule, and she knows that if she does not work in a swift and efficient manner, she will fall further and further behind as the morning goes on. As she prepares Mrs. Smith for her bath, she notices a change in Mrs. Smith's manner. Normally quite talkative, today she is quiet and rather distant. Joan, unfastening Mrs. Smith's gown, cautiously asks, "Mrs. Smith, how are you feeling today?"

No response.

"Didn't you sleep well last night?"

Mrs. Smith grudgingly mumbles something, so Joan continues her questioning of Mrs. Smith in an effort to find out what is bothering her. Joan is sitting beside the bed when Grace comes in the room. She notices that Joan is talking, not working.

"You have work to do, Joan, hurry up. Baths, the beds, and all treatments have to be finished. Talking this way is causing you to fall *really* behind." Grace turns and walks out.

Joan, feeling that Mrs. Smith needs her attention, stays with her until she confides her problem.

Joan's feelings of responsibility for her patient run counter to Grace's need for getting the work done; it is Joan who pays the price. Her next assignment might entail taking care of the most difficult patient.

Planning, scheduling, execution, and follow-up tell us how she does it, but the real key to understanding a 9,1-oriented head nurse's approach is to be found in communication and conflict.

COMMUNICATION

Clarity of communication is important to ensure that everything is understood. The nursing administrator spells out what is expected—a, b, c. . . . "These are your instructions. Unless you have questions, that's all for now."

The formula followed is, "Tell 'em, tell 'em you told 'em, and then tell 'em again." That's efficiency. There is little or no need for the staff to ask questions of the administrator whose instructions are clear and thorough because they increase her certainty that she is fully understood. Questions may tell her something else, and that is that the staff nurses have not been listening. Even more threatening, questions may mean that someone is not convinced; therefore the question challenges her authority.

Sometimes staff members will ask questions rather than express disagreement on what is being discussed. If these questions continue, the 9,1-oriented nurse's put-down is the use of sarcasm to make the person asking the question appear stupid. Repeated questions imply resistance or insubordination. The nursing administrator herself does not seek information, much less advice or opinion, from staff members as this would indicate weakness on her part. Having to ask implies that she does not know and therefore is not on top of things.

An example of "clear" communication of orders comes through in the following where we see Helen, head nurse, conducting a weekly staff meeting to tell her staff what is going on.

After the weekly meeting led by the director of nurses, Helen bustles into the conference room, having called a meeting with her own staff. She considers this a good way of keeping them informed, but it is usually one-way communication.

Helen speaks. "I want to tell you what went on in today's meeting. We have fifteen minutes so I have to hurry. The lab is coming out with a new form, so be sure all parts are filled in before sending it down or they won't take the blood. Also, next Monday Barbara Kramer is coming as a guest speaker. This is important, so I expect all of you to be there."

Ginny, a staff nurse, holds up her hand, "Helen, about those forms . . ."

"I said we only had fifteen minutes," Helen cuts in. "Ask me later after you've seen a copy. However, you should be able to figure it out."

On the way out of the room, Ginny nudges another staff nurse, "If I have any questions I'll ask you. I don't want to face her more than twice a day!"

This kind of communicating on an "ask-me-no-questions" basis does little more than alert the staff to potential problems. It is insufficient to help effect implementation in a way that can happen when people are clear as to what is expected of them.

The primary reaction by the staff nurse to one-way communication from the nursing administrator is compliance, but often with inward reservations. As staff members learn that the way to stay out of trouble is to obey, they are likely to follow the letter of the message, even though they may know a better way or even know that something will go wrong. When useful information available to the staff nurse is withheld, "Why didn't you tell me?" is answered with, "You didn't ask."

Another example of the nursing administrator being a link in the communication chain is in connection with doctors' written directions regarding medication or new orders that are written during the morning rounds. In the following situation, Carolyn, the head nurse, fails to alert Sue, the staff nurse, as to Mr. Kaplan's medication.

Carolyn, head nurse, is making morning rounds with Dr. Williams. They enter Mr. Kaplan's room. Dr. Williams, scanning Mr. Kaplan's chart, asks, "How are you this morning?" Mr. Kaplan grimaces a little as he touches his leg. "I'm still having pain in my knee. The nurse tells me she doesn't have a medication order."

Carolyn glances at Dr. Williams. "It just ran out this morning, doctor."

"No problem, Mr. Kaplan," Dr. Williams replies consolingly, "I'll write a new one. You should get something now and every four hours if you need it."

As they leave the room, Mr. Kaplan raises his hand to say goodbye. "Thanks, doctor. Other than that everything is okay."

"Good," Dr. Williams responds. "I'll see you tomorrow."

Dr. Williams goes out to the desk and writes the order.

Carolyn is on her way to find Mr. Kaplan's nurse, Sue. At that moment, she is approached by Jack, an LPN, who tells her that a patient in the lounge is having trouble breathing. Carolyn hurries off to the lounge and forgets to tell Sue about the medication order.

An hour later, Mr. Kaplan's wife approaches Carolyn in the hall and is furious. "My husband has been waiting, in pain, for two hours to receive some medication. Can you tell me why he hasn't?"

Carolyn is immediately angered too, more at herself because she is beginning to feel the pressures closing in on her. When she does find Sue, her anger is unleashed, and she yells, "Why don't you check your patient orders more frequently? I can't do everything around here!"

The real problem in the preceding situation is Carolyn's concept of herself as an administrator, seeing herself as indispensable to the unit, even to overseeing the smallest detail. She has little time to deal with unanticipated situations or touch base with Sue. She is unaware of this, however, and believes the problem is that Sue is not keeping up with new orders.

A nursing administrator communicates with other personnel who contribute to patient services; for example, x-ray and lab technicians, dietitians, and therapists. She has to inform her staff about preop medication orders, and sometimes postop orders are given staff nurses on the patient's return from the recovery room. These kinds of communications go through the nursing administrator, either into her unit from other departments or from her unit to other departments.

CONFLICT

Conflict is inevitable when persons who work together have feelings about what is right or wrong, good or bad, or sound or unsound. A 9,1-oriented nurse feels that she is losing control when conflict occurs, for her will is not being carried out when others question it, complain, or fail to toe the mark.

Anger is her reaction to the frustrations that result when someone does not comply. The anger, once aroused, does not go away; it persists and smolders and becomes more intense as she broods on it even though the original cause that may have aroused it has been reduced or eliminated. When this goes on for any length of time, the 9,1-oriented nursing administrator is likely to develop a surplus of anger and hostility, with the result that she constantly looks for excuses to vent anger on others. Sometimes this "free-floating" anger becomes so routine that others may see her as carrying a chip on her shoulder.

When conflict does erupt, suppression is the preferred way to deal with it in order to restore a sense of control. Suppression means that the other person is denied any chance to react.

Mistakes and errors

Sometimes, in spite of the head nurse's best efforts to be clear and direct, things do go wrong. Mistakes are made, errors occur, people blunder. Mistakes usually mean that people either were not working as they should, or they were making something go wrong on purpose. An incident report is written when an error is made, and this ultimately goes to hospital administration. This is considered a black mark on a nursing administrator's record.

Mistakes and errors can be found in many places. The wrong dosage can be ordered by the doctor and go unchallenged by the staff nurse even though she knows it is wrong. Some patients fall out of bed, particularly "sundowners." They have a knack for removing the restraints that have been put on them. Others may even fall out of the wheelchair as they slip down and out of their restraints. All of these are considered mistakes and errors on the part of the staff.

The question is, how does a 9,1-oriented nursing administrator deal with mistakes? Whether the error is written up or not, she never willingly overlooks a mistake. She cannot put up with an error in any form. Why? Because she knows if it happens once, it will happen again. Her immediate reaction on finding a mistake is "Who did it? This calls for disciplinary action." She carries out an inquisition to force the staff member in question to admit fault, allowing no excuses or explanations that might explain why something went wrong. Any rationalization or explanation is suppressed.

"Here is what you did wrong. Don't let it happen again or I will have to take disciplinary action."

The following is an example of a 9,1-oriented head nurse's way of dealing with mistakes. Jo Ann, head nurse, immediately seeks out the person responsible for the error and angrily jumps on Debra, staff nurse, decreeing that it should never happen again.

Dr. Wheeler briskly walks up to the nurse's station and lays his patients' charts on the corner of the head nurse's desk. Going through the pile of charts, he pulls one out and says, "Mr. File seems unusually sleepy this morning. I can't arouse him. What medication did he receive last night?"

Jo Ann, the head nurse, takes Mr. File's chart and notes that he was given a Nembutal at 1 a.m. this morning.

"Nembutal? Who gave him that? I certainly didn't order it for him." Dr. Wheeler's color begins to rise as he points the questions at Jo Ann, who has already noted that Debra was on duty last night.

"I'm sorry, doctor, this is terrible. I'll see that it doesn't happen again." She quickly turns and hurries down the hall, her indignation and anger only visible by her jaw set in clenched teeth. "Of all the stupid . . . What in the world was Debra thinking about to do a dumb thing like that?" she thinks. She backtracks to the nurse's station and picks up the phone, dialing Debra's number. "Debbie?" Jo Ann can hardly control her voice. "Dr. Wheeler and I have discovered you mistakenly gave Mr. File a Nembutal last night. I don't know or care to know how it happened; you just make sure you fill out an incident report when you come on duty tonight. And I don't want to *ever* hear of your making a dumb mistake like that again!" She slams down the phone in anger.

On the other end of the line, Debbie groggily puts the phone back on the hook and wonders if she is having a bad dream.

Jo Ann's manner of dealing with this situation gives Debra no opportunity to explore the circumstances surrounding the error in order to learn why it happened and thus be in a better position to avoid a similar mistake in the future. It does give Jo Ann a sense of power, however, but her method of assigning blame and using threat will ultimately only create negative attitudes and antagonism toward her.

Mistakes and errors are seen as arising from bad attitudes. Disciplinary action is used to prevent them from being repeated. These kinds of retributions by the nursing administrator lead to at least two reactions on the part of the staff—fear and resentment. If a staff member is sufficiently fearful of the head nurse, she may become a bundle of nerves, so tense that she is all thumbs and can possibly even admit doing things wrong when she did not. Alternatively, the staff nurse becomes so resentful that every time the head nurse says, "You did it," the staff nurse says back (at least to herself) "I didn't." Out of sheer defiance she refuses to admit anything. She and the head nurse come to a standoff, at least on the surface.

This way of dealing with mistakes can result in the staff causing even more mistakes. Yet few real perpetrators get caught. Staff members go underground with errors. Incident reports are not written, which also can lead to unfortunate results. As mistakes reappear, those who cause them remain hidden. Many times the head nurse will never know "who did it."

Complaints

Complaints relating to the character of work take the form of: "The equipment doesn't work correctly." "There is no more linen—we've run out of it." "We've worked so much overtime we're tired." After a while, these mount up and the head nurse finally hears them. How does a 9,1-oriented nursing administrator deal with complaints?

Her basic attitude is to see them as a lack of strength, or at least as an indication of weakness. She ignores, belittles, or bullies those who complain.

"Don't bother me with your complaints. If you're doing your job, you won't have the time or inclination to gripe."

The 9,1-oriented nursing administrator passes off a complaint by using any of the following suppression tactics. She says, "If you don't like it here, leave." or "Go tell it to someone else." She may simply put it back on the staff member and say, "It's really a rough world for everybody. Quit complaining."

She can bully her staff member by saying, "Stop being a crybaby." All of these suppression tactics say to the complainer, "You've never had it so good if that's all you've go to complain about."

The attitude, in other words, is that if she listens to complaints, she is open to a never-ending round of griping. She runs the risk of becoming a counseling center. Then she would never have any time to get out the work. The way to deal with complaints is to brush them aside, or to make the complainer ashamed of wasting her time bringing up something of such little importance.

This way of suppressing complaints has repercussions down the line and even is felt by patients. Staff nurses who are not listened to become frustrated and, when a patient complains, deliver the same treatment to the patient. The patient is ignored and complaints go on deaf ears. Because of these reactions, patients soon learn not to complain. Even if the patients' families complain about the care patients receive, patients are not always happy because they know there may possibly be repercussions.

For this reason complaints are sometimes not known about until the patient goes home. The patient goes home and subsequently sends a letter to the hospital. The patient's family member writes the director of nurses or the administrator regarding poor care or the negative attitudes of the staff. If these sources of complaints are eventually relayed to the head nurse, then the heat is felt by the staff and the frustration and tensions mount even more. The following is an example.

Nora Washington, director of nurses at Memorial Hospital, looks through the mail her secretary has opened. One in particular catches her eye:

Dear Ms. Washington:

This letter is to convey to you my dissatisfaction with the care I received while a patient in Room 201, 3 West June 10-15. As you know I had some complications after my surgery and there were numerous times when I rang the nurses and no one came. On the average your staff nurses were rude when they did attend me.

One other thing. I felt it absolutely unnecessary for nurses' aids, interns, and other such persons to come into my room unannounced. There were times I felt like a guinea pig, and I resented it very much.

In the future, should I or any of my family have to go into the hospital, it will not be Memorial.

Sincerely,

Carla Jones

Nora picks up the phone and asks Janice, the head nurse on the unit, to come to her office. She lets her read Carla Jones' letter. By the time she is finished, Janice explodes, "This is the first time I've heard about it! But I have told my staff time and time again that they are here to take care of the patient. I'm going right now and find out who is responsible." And she does, venting her wrath upon anyone and everyone who was near Carla Jones during her stay.

A vicious cycle is set up. The head nurse does not listen to the staff's complaints; the staff will not always listen to the patient's complaints. When patients have been labeled as complainers, or as difficult to get along with, a staff nurse does not want to take care of them. So if the food is cold, the bath is poorly given, the bell is not answered quickly, or the patient wets the bed and is not changed quickly, these are ways the staff nurse gets back at the patient because this is how the head nurse treats the staff.

In the following example, Sue, head nurse, cuts short any protest regarding the pressure and long hours that Lee, the staff nurse, is experiencing.

This is one of those nights when a large number of emergency patients have been admitted to the coronary care unit. Sue is really concerned about the care of her patients. In addition, several patients have had cardiac arrests. Staff nurses have been working at a high pace and have not had a chance to take a coffee break or be relieved.

When Lee White, staff nurse, sees Sue approaching, Lee says, "I haven't had a break in ages. I'm about to drop."

Sue replies, "Well, this is what you're here for and you've just got to work." When Lee balks, Sue says, "You know this is a specialized unit. There are not many people who can be 'floated' in to relieve us. Don't expect anything better. If you don't like it, you can leave. But for now, don't let me hear any more about it."

Sue is so concerned about the patients, she could not care less at this moment about how Lee White is holding up. She intensifies Lee's tensions by adding to them, leaving her with the feeling of certainty that she is being taken advantage of. Her complaints become hostile feelings that become seething resentment.

Hostile feelings

Many staff nurses become frustrated and resentful working day after day under a 9,1-oriented nursing administrator. If the staff nurse tells the nursing administrator what she thinks in a hostile or provocative way, the 9,1-oriented nursing administrator reacts to her in such a way as to turn it into a win-lose argument or an open fight. Her attitude is:

"Negative attitudes are a sign of insubordination; people who act up are bad apples and the sooner I put them in their place the better."

Why is it important that hostile feelings be suppressed so promptly? Hostile feelings expressed toward the head nurse or director of nurses are unacceptable because, under a 9,1 orientation, authority is the backbone for achieving results through people. Hostile feelings undermine the nursing administrator's capacity for exercising her authority. They have a bad effect on production, which cannot be tolerated. If they persist, her worst fear is that the system will break down, showing her up as a failure.

When hostile feelings manifest themselves in a fight or win-lose argument, they tend to persist and become chronic even after the argument is resolved. Every time the head nurse, in a gruff or nonconciliatory way, says, "Cool it," staff members say, at least to themselves, "Drop dead." When hostile behavior persists, the 9,1-oriented nursing administrator seeks to arrange a transfer for the staff nurse to get her out of her hair. She gives her problem child to someone else.

For the nursing staff a sour note in their relationship with a 9,1-oriented nursing administrator is her arrogance. This source of friction, however, is not likely to come out into the open. The staff's frustrations toward her are expressed behind her back, in gripe sessions or even with others outside the unit. Unfortunately, expressing frustrations does little or nothing to relieve them.

In the following example, Victoria, the 9,1-oriented head nurse, reprimands Mary, staff nurse, for taking time out to talk with Mr. Grasso, an upset patient. Mary snaps back indignantly to Victoria, who in turn sets her straight regarding her hostile attitudes.

Victoria, the head nurse in a forty-bed med-surg unit, is sitting at the nurses' station reviewing doctor order sheets. It is 10:30 a.m. and doctors have started making their rounds.

Mary, one of the staff nurses, comes up to the desk and inquires, "Are there any orders for Mr. Forrest in 203?" Victoria begins looking for Mr. Forrest's sheet and then glares up at Mary. "You mean you haven't seen him yet?"

"No," says Mary, slightly flushing, "I've been with Mr. Grasso half the morning. He had several questions about his illness and seems rather upset today."

"But Mary," Victoria says heatedly, "you're behind in your assignments. You know that on this unit we complete our work by eleven. You're wasting time talking with patients. Get those procedures done and the blood pressures taken!"

"But Ms. Rose," Mary replies with conviction, "I think listening to the patient . . ."

". . . is the doctor's job, not yours," retorts Victoria.

"I didn't take a coffee break, Ms. Rose," Mary comes back heatedly. "Mr. Grasso was so upset. Someone needs to listen so that . . ."

Victoria interrupts, ". . . so that he'll learn that complaining gets attention. Oh no, that's not your responsibility, and I'll thank you not to talk back to me. Also, Mary, I understand you've stayed overtime talking to patients without authorization. I can't have that kind of thing going on; it just messes up the whole unit. Let's get on schedule, shall we?"

Mary, flushed, hurriedly goes off in the direction of Mr. Forrest's room.

Victoria, who sees "talking" to patients as a waste of time, reprimands Mary and sees her efforts as insubordination since she is failing to carry out orders. Victoria cuts off Mary's attempts to justify her actions and sends her back to work. We can imagine that Mary will not spread joy over the unit today, and Mr. Forrest suffers the most as he is the next one in line. The cycle goes like this: Victoria unloads on Mary, Mary unloads on Mr. Forrest, Mr. Forrest unloads on his wife, his wife unloads on the doctor . . .

DEVELOPMENT

Because the 9,1-oriented nursing administrator is so task oriented, she is very interested in getting the job done. This means that her personnel have to be very strong; they have to know what they are supposed to be doing and not need to ask questions. Therefore, as far as orientation goes, she sees to it that her staff becomes oriented to the unit so that they will not have any questions about who is boss, what they are supposed to do, and how the procedures are to be administered. She has a planned program, again so that there is no need for questions, no need for deviations from the procedures as she administers them.

"I get strong people and weed out the weak ones. What they get in inservice is still okay, but I concentrate on staff nurses learning on the job so that I know it is done right."

In the following example, Sylvia, head nurse, knows that Sally will get all she needs to know by studying the procedures used on her unit. If Sally has trouble, it is because she is inattentive or does not put forth effort.

Sally is a new staff nurse assigned to Sylvia's unit. After Sally had gone through orientation in the inservice department, the supervisor brought her to the unit and introduced her to Sylvia.

"Welcome to our unit, Sally. One of the first things I have my staff do is read the policy and procedure manuals. Go over these and I'll check back with you later." Sylvia looks at her watch and leaves.

Sally scans the thick manual with dismay. "All of these?" she murmurs to herself, "I hope I don't have to memorize them. I did hear she's a drill sergeant . . ."

A little later Sylvia returns and continues the discussion. "These policies and procedures provide the guidelines for how I run my unit, which is a clean, tight ship. We will get along fine if you carry out the assignments as I make them. That way fewer mistakes are made. So if you have any questions come to me direct. Now, let's go out on the floor and I'll show you around. Please listen carefully as I explain our routine because I don't have time to repeat myself. Ready? Let's go."

Sylvia moves off quickly without waiting for Sally to reply.

As the weeks go by, Sally struggles to do what is expected. After her "orientation" she knows better than to ask questions. If things don't fall into place easily she would rather try to find out what to do from other staff members than to suffer Sylvia's barbs.

This is a 9,1 orientation to development because it tells staff members directly what to do without exceptions and without any questions asked. Since a head nurse who operates in this way rarely is asked any questions and yet sees evidence of violations and mistakes, she assumes that staff members are lazy and really do not want to work. After a preliminary orientation to rules and procedures, a 9,1 orientation contains at least two ideas for inducting the staff member. One is this:

"The best way to measure a staff nurse's caliber is to throw her in the thick of it. The strong ones will swim and the weaker sink. There's not much you can do better than to put a nurse to the acid test. You might as well find out what you've got and quick."

The 9,1-oriented nursing administrator also relies on performance evaluations to indicate to a staff nurse what is going wrong. She uses her power to give poor ratings as both punishment for misbehavior and as a threat to motivate greater effort. For a staff nurse who is giving trouble there will be more frequent performance reviews, from one per year to one every ninety days, or every sixty days, or even more often, building up pressure until the staff member has shaped up to meet the nursing administrator's wishes. Each time there are remarks about the annual evaluation that is drawing nearer and nearer. "You've really slumped this month, and it's going to show at your next evaluation. You had better pull yourself together."

Evidently Jill, staff nurse in the following example, is performing well, but Nona, head nurse, recognizes only outstanding performance. "Otherwise a nurse might let up."

Jill is sitting at the nurses' station waiting for her evaluation with the head nurse, Nona. Jill has been on 3 South a year this week. As this is her first real evaluation since being employed here, she is understandably nervous, not so much about the evaluation itself but because of Nona. She is a real slave driver.

Nona approaches and pulls her chair up beside Jill's. "Look, Jill," she begins. "This should only take a few minutes. I know you are busy, and I certainly have things to do." She pulls out the evaluation sheet and glances over it. "The first thing I want to say to you is that I rarely give above 'satisfactory' evaluations. There are few nurses who reach my standards. It appears you are doing okay, but there is always room for improvement."

Jill's first reaction is to protest. But then she hesitates. "What's the use? I know Nona well enough to know that whatever I say will fall on deaf ears."

Nona's 9,1-oriented approach is "Here is the way I see it; now all you have to do is improve. Period." No discussion, really, and no opportunity for Jill to object.

CHANGE BY EDICT

The onrush of technology and of new thinking about better ways of administration creates the certainty that change occurs at least at a steady pace, or, in all probability, at an ever-increasing rate. Additional pressures for change are from government regulations regarding such items as cost control and funding.

Because the 9,1-oriented nursing administrator is in charge, she may be intensely pressuring for change to correct the situation as she sees it. Change requirements are *imposed* on those who report to her. This is likely to provide active or underground resistance and resentment from those who are to implement the change.

A 9,1-oriented director of nurses or head nurse ramrods proposed changes into effect. In the following example, the director of nurses, Laura Cole, is convinced that the unit manager form of organization is ideal for her hospital.

She clears her intended administrative setup with the hospital administrator, who has long since learned not to oppose her proposals.

On Friday, Laura Cole calls a special meeting with her head nurses and announces, "It has been decided that we will shift our organization practices starting Monday morning from our current approach to the unit manager system. We can't do this all at once, but starting on Monday we will make the shiftover first in your unit, Sue. The unit manager has already been hired and will report for work Monday morning. His name is Smith. He is retired Army. Other units will be shifted as unit managers can be employed."

Silence falls on the meeting as Laura terminates her announcement, but it is by no means an easy silence. After a period of time questions begin to arise: "What is this unit manager going to do?" "Who is going to train him?" "You said that the unit manager is going to take care of the order book, replace broken equipment, take responsibility for housekeeping. What do you expect me to do?" Laura responds to these kinds of queries in an accusative way saying, "These are all matters of administration that you have been complaining about and I am relieving you of these responsibilities in one fell swoop. That's what will be so wonderful about the unit manager system."

Sue asks, "Does this mean that he will be sitting with me at my station?"

Laura replies, "No, two people at a desk is not very efficient and only creates an environment where people interrupt one another and get in the way of good performance. We'll set up a desk for Mr. Smith on the other side."

Smith arrives on Monday morning and an immediate clash of personalities is evident. The head nurse and Smith become enemies, and the director of nurses, Laura, feeling that her unit manager plan hangs in the balance, decides to resolve the conflict by dismissing the head nurse, Sue.

Though not made explicit, the general reactions of the head nurses are seething resentment at a unilateral decision having been made and announced for application without any preparation or consultation or discussion or thinking through. Issues of compatibility have been ignored, and it can be anticipated that the head nurses, feeling threatened, will not be motivated to help Mr. Smith but rather to create conditions under which his performance will look bad.

This example of a 9,1 way of bringing change into existence demonstrates the adverse impact from change by edict. Those whose lives are affected by the change resisted, not because of any fundamental resistance to change, but rather because of the arbitrary manner in which the change was introduced.

REACTIONS TO 9,1 SUPERVISION

The day-to-day influences and effects from 9,1-oriented supervision have been identified. However, there are longer-term implications of this approach that also need to be identified and understood.

The complaint reaction

It is well known in hospitals that some staff nurses not only expect to be supervised in a 9,1 manner, but that they *enjoy* the routine of being told explicitly what to do, when to do it, and then what to do next. This staff nurse is not a self-mover but a compliant individual who is prepared to execute rather than to think.

All goes well with the daily routine when a unit is administered in a 9,1-oriented manner and staffed by nurses in this compliant orientation. The difficulties arise, however, when crises appear. When important actions need to be taken and there is no one immediately available to say who should take what initiative, or even to authorize what the nurse already knows should be done, the system breaks down. It is then that chaos prevails and unfortunate consequences result.

Resentment and insurrection

At the opposite extreme from dutiful compliance is the reaction of many staff nurses whose feelings of professionalism are violated when told in an authoritarian manner what they should be doing and how to do it. They feel that demands are placed upon them that are arbitrary, excessive, and sometimes constitute intrusions into their private lives. When a unit is staffed by nurses who feel antipathy and resentment toward the nursing administrator, the attitude is "Let the head nurse suffer." The most unanticipated results may occur. All of a sudden there is a sit-down, even a walk-out, or at the very least an insistent demand that corrective actions be taken before further nursing services will be provided. This often comes as a great surprise and shock to the nursing administrator, who is likely to feel that all of her efforts in behalf of patients have evaporated and she is unappreciated.

The withdrawal reaction

A third reaction can occur on a unit when nurses are unprepared to be compliant but are not in a position to feel secure or confident in fighting back. These are often nurses whose husbands need the additional support that the wife's employment can provide, or whose families make it necessary to work, and leave the nurses little or no option other than to take it. These are the ones who withdraw into a shell and in this way escape the pressures, tensions, frustrations, and antagonisms that they otherwise would experience. By dehumanizing the situation, they avoid the frustrations of living and working in a system that violates their professionalism and personal integrity. The result is that they contribute the minimum necessary to stay out of trouble, and withhold any exercise of initiative, even when the need for it is obvious and self-evident. These are the nurses who are likely to earn the label of "lazy." They are not lazy, but simply resentful and express this resentment by walking away from the job while staying on it.

Leaving

Being unable to rectify the situation through confrontation of the 9,1-oriented nursing administrator, or the use of feedback and critique to help her to see the consequences of her modes of administration, many staff nurses are not in a situation where they have to take it any longer. The consequence is that they leave. This is done in several ways. Some leave through advancement and become nursing administrators themselves, vowing never to supervise others as they have been supervised, but frequently slipping into the very trap that their acceptance of advancement had been calculated to resolve. Some leave by taking staff nurse assignments in other units that are supervised in a better way. Some, unfortunately, leave the profession of nursing entirely, unprepared to continue under unattractive and unpleasant circumstances. This consequence of 9,1 supervision is probably the most cited reason for nurses leaving the profession today.

SUMMARY

The 9,1-oriented nursing administrator concentrates on planning and scheduling, execution, and follow-up. She thinks out what her staff nurses should be doing and when they should be doing it. More than that, she keeps checking to ensure that things go as she intends. By doing these things, she relies on no one but herself. This way she is in charge; she alone is responsible. Her assumption is that high production will result from her thoroughness, her attention to detail, her keeping on top of each activity as it occurs, and her negative evaluations of those who fail to measure up.

Communication is done on an "ask-me-no-questions" basis. The nursing administrator spells out what is to be expected with great clarity so that everything is understood and thereby the need for any questions to be asked is eliminated.

The staff basically cannot be trusted. Too many things can go wrong if the nursing administrator is not checking and double-checking. After all, mistakes, errors, and complaints reflect badly on her supervision. They indicate to her superiors that she is not in control of things. If things really get bad this suggests that she is a failure and cannot bring it off.

Over a period of time, staff nurses supervised by a 9,1-oriented head nurse or director of nurses learn that there is no room for the exercise of autonomy and independent judgment in completing one's professional responsibilities. When emergencies arise, they either wait until someone else recognizes them or a staff nurse seeks out the head nurse for advice and authorization as to what should be done.

For newly hired staff members, a 9,1-oriented nursing administrator has a planned program so that there will be no need for deviations from the procedures as she administers them. Performance evaluation is a way of rewarding performers and punishing nonperformers.

Any change is introduced into the organization by edict.

Therefore, we see that the 9,1-oriented nursing administrator who on the surface of things may run an efficient medical service is more frequently than not creating the conditions under which patients will receive less-than-adequate care.

Chapter 4

THE 1,9-ORIENTED NURSING ADMINISTRATOR

A 1,9-oriented nursing administrator is characterized by geniality; she seeks to be friendly to everyone. Harmony comes from showering the staff with kindness, being aware of the progress of the children and relatives, showing an active interest in a vacation trip, and so on. She pays attention to those who are left out and lonely, seeking to create a climate of approval with compliments and positive reactions to specific requests. Work is enjoyable and life more pleasant with an appreciative pat on the back, a smile, a cup of coffee. This creates an attitude of sharing, a sense of warmth, mutuality, a balm of security. She courts the acceptance and approval of others by extending acceptance and approval to them. Such acts of endorsement promote community and ward off the potentially disgruntled staff member who might otherwise express unhappiness.

The 1,9-oriented nursing administrator wants to be approved of and accepted so that she feels comfortable, secure, and happy in her work. Her way of gaining acceptance is through doing whatever is asked of her by doctors and those above her in a warm and responsive way. She approaches her staff members in much the same manner, seeking always to be pleasant and friendly and doing her best to avoid putting pressure on them. Whenever problems arise, she is ready to pitch in and offer help, and in this way reduce any sense of frustration that others might otherwise feel toward her. Even though she is the boss, her tendency is to defer to the wishes of others, regardless of whether these are in the line of duty.

Sometimes a 1,9-oriented nursing administrator fails to receive the warmth and approval she wants, no matter how hard she may try. Her greatest fear is to suffer rejection, to sense that others may not like her or what it is that she is obligated to ask of them. When rejection does occur, it is very disturbing and increases her feeling of insecurity and uncertainty. Her way of trying to restore acceptance and warmth is to placate and apologize and promise, "Next time, I will be more thoughtful and will do my best to prevent this situation from happening again."

In summary, to be accepted is what a 1,9-oriented nursing administrator most strives to realize; being disliked and suffering rejection is what she seeks most to avoid.

Now we can study how these motivations become evident in her approach to the supervision of her own staff.

An acceptant environment is all-important. After all, when she and her staff nurses are on a warm and friendly basis, the situation is intrinsically enjoyable. Even beyond that, they are thoughtful and helpful to one another. It then becomes unnecessary to push people, as they "know" the importance of doing the best they can. Therefore, the 1,9-oriented nursing administrator makes every effort to establish good relationships. She works on how to get them, how to keep them, what to do to keep them from going sour, and how to restore good relationships whenever tensions arise.

NURSE IN THE MIDDLE

As far as a 1,9-oriented nursing administrator is concerned, her loyalty lies with her staff. However, on a one-to-one basis with the director of nurses, doctors, and anyone else outside her unit for that matter, she maintains a willing-to-please manner. Whatever is asked of her, she does, oftentimes in the most literal sense, as it is often better to do a task herself rather than to ask someone else and risk their displeasure.

If new procedures, policies, or regulations occur, her first reaction is, "What will my staff think? Will they complain?" If she feels that the changes will anger or frustrate any of them, she may even delay telling them. When she does tell them and they do not like it, then it is she and her staff against the administration. "They won't let me do it." After all, it is the staff's welfare she is concerned about; it is important that they are a part of a pleasant work setting. When she is with her supervisors, on the other hand, she embraces what "they" want.

Torn between keeping her staff happy and maintaining good relationships with her superiors and the doctors sometimes has its strains, but it is worth it; her reward is comments like, "I enjoy working on this unit; there's no pressure." "We're just one happy family."

From a director of nurses' perspective, it is important to maintain a harmonious relationship with the hospital administrator and the nurses she supervises, not particularly to make the hospital run more efficiently, but for her own personal need to be accepted and appreciated. This is her primary motivation, although she may not realize it herself.

In the following situation, Lanell Black, director of nurses, concentrates on smoothing out relationships and keeping everyone happy rather than trying to find out the root cause of the problem.

Rachel, head nurse, has asked for a few minutes to meet with Lanell to discuss a personnel situation that she is facing in her unit.

"They are both very competent nurses," Rachel is saying. "As far as doing their work is concerned, I couldn't ask for any better people. But they simply can't get along. Their attitudes can't help but affect others; even the patients notice it. There are times when you can cut the air with a knife. Somehow I have a feeling Jane feels hostile toward Beth because she has a BS degree. I don't really know. There's something between them I can't seem to put by finger on. I'm hoping you will talk to them; I can't seem to get a handle on it myself."

Lanell agrees to talk to the two staff nurses. She decides to have both in at the same time. She schedules a time for ten o'clock, and both of them arrive in her office on time. Jane and Beth sit stiffly in their chairs, waiting for Lanell to speak.

Lanell clears her throat nervously and smiles, "Well, I hear you two are having some difficulty." Neither Jane nor Beth responds. The silence is heavy and perspiration breaks out on Lanell's forehead. She feebly begins again, "Listen, why don't you two patch things up. After all, you have good jobs here—good pay and benefits—it's no fun not getting along. I tell you what, why don't you both take an hour off early today. Maybe that will make you feel better. Then tomorrow everything will be forgotten."

Beth starts to say something and then decides against it. Jane merely drops her eyes and nods her head as if to say, "Whatever you say." Lanell takes this as a sign of agreement. "Good!" she exclaims, "Now let's go to the lounge and have some coffee."

In Lanell's eyes, all is well. But the tension between Jane and Beth still exists. Lanell's effort was to create warm and friendly feelings. Her thought was that if they had a pleasant time socially, they would learn to like one another. This may only temporarily suspend ill feelings, but no doubt Rachel will visit Lanell again with the same complaint.

ADMINISTRATIVE ASPECTS OF NURSING

The production requirements of patient care are revealed in 1,9-oriented attitudes toward planning and scheduling, execution, and follow-up.

Planning and scheduling

The daily activities of a 1,9-oriented nursing administrator are the same as under any other Grid style. The time has to be kept, assignments have to be made, and scheduling must be done. The difference is that she avoids pressuring her staff members, preferring rather to let each person operate on her own after initial instructions are given. In other words, her attitude is:

"Even though it's not possible to please everyone, I try to ensure that my staff members are given assignments that they like best."

The 1,9-oriented nursing administrator wants her unit to be a pleasant and comfortable place to work. If at all possible, coffee times and lunch periods are usually taken at personal preference. The shift schedule is often maneuvered to fit individual desires.

In the following situation, Natalie, head nurse, finds herself in the dilemma of how to cover her unit and meet a request for time off from Rita, her staff nurse.

Natalie is straightening the linen closet when Rita, one of the youngest nurses on her unit, comes in. "Natalie, I can hardly keep my mind on my work today; it's such a beautiful spring day. My boyfriend just called and wants to drive up to the lake this afternoon. Do you think I could take off an hour early?"

Natalie can't help but think of the full patient load they are experiencing; practically every room on the unit is full, and several patients are seriously ill. Yet she knows how Rita feels—it is a gorgeous day and somehow she couldn't risk Rita being unhappy. "I hate to tell her no," she thinks, "maybe I can work something out." "Well, I don't see why you can't, Rita," she says. "You go ahead and have a good time."

"Thanks, Natalie!" Rita hurriedly leaves the room, eager to tell the other staff nurses about her plans. Patient care has already left her mind.

Natalie stacks the last of the sheets on the shelf. "I'll just cover for her somehow," she muses. "After all, Rita is a good worker."

Here we see Natalie's concern for keeping Rita happy overshadowing her concern for administering patient care. The result is that someone will have to assume Rita's duties for the rest of the day. It is unlikely that Natalie will ask another staff nurse to pick up the assignment. Natalie is more likely to do it herself. In any event, a hardship will be placed on someone in the name of promoting harmony and goodwill.

Execution

The 1,9-oriented nursing administrator gives staff members freedom in carrying out assignments rather than giving detailed directions. Her attitude might be as follows:

"I give broad assignments to my staff and convey my confidence by saying, 'I'm sure you know how to do this and you will do it well.'"

One of the dilemmas in any hospital unit is the supervision of the staff nurses who constantly put their personal needs above the needs of their patients. In the following example, Michelle, staff nurse on 8 West, cannot quite get it together to carry out one of her assignments for that day. Grace is the head nurse on that unit.

Michelle groans as she slowly walks down the hall to the nurse's station. She puts her hand to her head, hoping the coolness of it will relieve the throbbing she feels in her right temple. "I ought to know better than to go dancing on a week night. How will I ever get through this day? And this afternoon I'm supposed to do patient teaching with Ms.

Gold. She goes home tomorrow morning and she's been so upset since her colostomy. Oh, well, I'm too tired to think about it. Maybe Grace will do it for me. She's good about covering for us."

"Well, good morning," Grace says warmly, as Michelle approaches. "You look tired and it's only seven in the morning!"

"Grace, I stayed out too late last night and I feel awful. On top of that I have to teach Ms. Gold today."

"Well, sit down for a while and relax." Grace busies herself tidying up. "Besides," she continues, "Ms. Gold can wait. Her family can't pick her up until four this afternoon."

Michelle flops down and stretches out her legs. Yawning, she says, "Did you see 'Medical Journal' last Tuesday night on TV? Isn't Dr. Williams handsome!"

Grace is so concerned about Michelle that the importance of teaching Ms. Gold has suddenly diminished. Under this approach, assignments are often done in a slipshod manner, and there is usually a backlog of things to be done. It is not surprising in this instance that teaching Ms. Gold has been relegated to the last minute.

Follow-up

A 1,9-oriented nursing administrator avoids imposing her will on staff members. She supports rather than pushes. Therefore her attitude in checking on how and when assignments have been carried out might be put this way:

"I know my nurses try to do their best and I go out of my way to congratulate each one. I'm here to help and encourage them."

Actually, checking up on her staff is her least liked responsibility. Although she recognizes the fact that some nurses need closer supervision than others, she hesitates to do so. The prospect of conflict, hurt feelings, or even having to be unpleasant leaves her hoping that all things—all the time—run smoothly.

In the following example we see how Martha, head nurse, follows up with Jennifer, staff nurse, who has failed in her attempt to draw blood from a patient.

Jennifer is beginning to lose her patience. She cannot locate a vein in the arm of the patient, Paul Burns. She has tried twice, and now Mr. Burns is beginning to show his uneasiness. On Jennifer's third attempt, he asks exasperatedly, "Would you get someone who knows how to take blood!"

Jennifer hastily leaves the room. A few minutes later she returns with Martha, who immediately comforts Mr. Burns. "Don't you worry about a thing, Mr. Burns, we'll have you fixed up in a jiffy. It won't take me but a minute."

She quickly draws the blood sample, and, after seeing that Mr. Burns is comfortable, she and Jennifer leave the room. Martha consoles Jennifer by saying, "Don't worry about it. It has happened to me too. You just come get me when you think there is a problem." And she continues the conversation as they walk down the hall, making sure Jennifer suffers no hurt feelings and that she understands that Martha was there to help and support her.

Under this approach, any anxiety that Jennifer might have felt was relieved by Martha's "takeover" and her admonitions to not feel badly. Rather than teach Jennifer how to draw correctly, Martha focused on resolving the tensions Jennifer felt. No doubt throughout the day she also checked on Mr. Burns to make sure he too did not harbor any ill feelings.

COMMUNICATIONS

Because the key to understanding a nursing administrator's supervisory approach is seen through her actions as she communicates with others, and how she faces conflict, we will examine how a 1,9-oriented nurse will act under such circumstances.

A 1,9-oriented nursing administrator communicates frequently with all her staff. She wants to assure herself that everything is okay in the sense that people are feeling good. The best way she can do this is to stay in close, chatty conversation. Then she can detect any rumblings of unhappiness as they first begin to appear, or be helpful in assisting staff members to adjust to their situation, or take time to relieve whatever tensions may exist. This kind of conversation often is about topics that have nothing to do with work. A 1,9-oriented nursing administrator likes it even better if she can join a friendly discussion somebody else starts rather than take the initiative herself.

When she must give directions, a 1,9-oriented nursing administrator is likely to mention that a need exists, but she does so in an indirect way. She hopes that her staff will be interested enough to take the initiative themselves and to ask questions to find out more about the situation. In this way they will "own the problem." It is not imposed on them; rather it is picked up and now belongs to them. In this indirect manner, a 1,9-oriented nursing administrator seems always to be helping staff members to deal with their problems and almost never asks for their help in solving them.

Giving directions might be thought of as a general rather than a close kind of supervision, as is evident in the situation facing Karen, head nurse, in the following example.

Elizabeth Lewis, the supervisor of Karen's unit, is making rounds. Upon meeting Karen, Elizabeth says, "Karen, when is your staff going to start straightening up after themselves? The utility room is a mess—catheterization sets and other items are all over the place; bed pans are not emptied. What's going on?"

Karen, embarrassed, says, "When I meet with my staff today, I'll remind them."

Karen goes back to her station, wondering how she will bring up the subject with her staff. They have been getting on so well lately that she hates the thought of bringing up a problem. Besides that, they don't like Elizabeth either.

When eleven o'clock comes around, the staff, one by one, begins to gather around Karen's desk. She does not take part in their light conversation, and she thinks it terribly hot and stuffy today. Her uniform becomes almost sticky to her skin. Clearing her throat, she says awkwardly, "Listen, I hate to bring the subject up, but we are going to have to do more about improving the appearance of the utility room. Ms. Lewis was quite upset this morning."

Several hostile comments are heard, including, "We aren't paid to be maids. They ought to hire more aids." Karen feels very uncomfortable. All she can say is, "Well, I would appreciate whatever you can do about keeping the utility room neat."

Later in the day, when passing through the utility room, Karen notices that no one has done anything about straightening up, so trying not to be noticed, she begins to tidy up.

This is a 1,9-oriented approach to giving directions. When faced with rejection from her staff by bringing up an unpleasant subject, Karen backs off in a fashion that almost totally deemphasizes the importance of the request. Furthermore, anticipating the "moment of truth" when the director of nursing might check the utility room, she takes care of the problem herself.

This style of supervision certainly does not annoy people. Nor does it tie them down with self-defeating tensions or stimulate emotions that upset them. It does not even foster personal enmity toward the head nurse. It takes a "strong" 9,1 pusher to do that. Under 1,9-oriented supervision, staff members can work at whatever tempo is congenial and comfortable without fear that they will be taken to task for not doing more.

When it is necessary for her to ask questions of staff members, she is likely to do so by making them vague and general. In this way she avoids asking how things are going in a fashion that might annoy a staff nurse or appear to be prying, prodding, or critical of her work.

In the following example, Miriam, head nurse, fails to communicate to Nan, staff nurse, what has been brought to her attention as a violation of this particular hospital's policy of daily baths.

Miriam is seated at the nurse's station. She and Ella, LPN, are engaged in casual conversation as the early morning routine settles down to normalcy. The staff nurses are either at coffee or finishing up with patients. Ella is one of those persons who loves to chatter and spends a great deal of her time passing along tidbits of gossip that she overhears in the hospital. She is popular, especially with the patients, as she keeps everyone informed about everything.

Ella looks over Miriam's shoulder and says, "Hmmm, checking assignments. It looks like Nan gets through quicker than anyone." "Yes, she does," replies Miriam. "She's a very fast worker."

"Well, maybe I shouldn't say anything, but did you know that Nan only gives her patients baths every other day if she can get by with it? I've seen her initial her chart indicating a bath, but most of the time, if she's rushed, she'll skip it." Ella can't seem to talk fast enough now; the words rush out in a torrent. "She said not to mention it to you, but she couldn't really see what difference it makes."

Miriam's heart sinks. She knows that Nan is sloppy sometimes and is usually in a hurry to get through no matter what she is doing. But, maybe she can overlook this; after all, she has heard few complaints. Perhaps she will say something to Nan when she gets the opportunity.

Later, as Miriam enters the nurse's station, she sees Nan sitting there, thumbing through a magazine. "Look, Ms. Simpson, don't you think this is a great looking dress? I think I'll order it; after all, I deserve it!"

Miriam and Nan both laugh. In the back of her mind, Miriam remembers her promise to herself to bring up the skipped baths. "Oh, well," she thinks. "Maybe another day. This isn't the time."

This is a 1,9-oriented approach because Miriam does not want to risk creating tensions that might lead to feelings of rejection. By trying to keep her relationships with her staff on a harmonious basis, she is avoiding confronting those problems that are barriers to good patient care.

CONFLICT

Under a 1,9 orientation conflict is dreaded because it threatens warmth and approval, the main staples in the 1,9 emotional diet. This is what makes conflict seem so devastating. However, if conflict does arise, the nursing administrator tries to get back into a close supportive relationship as quickly as possible.

Mistakes and errors

No one likes mistakes and errors, least of all a 1,9-oriented nursing administrator. Her heart goes out to the person who has difficulties because she knows how badly that person must feel. Focusing on real or imagined "hurts" rather than on the mistake itself follows the 1,9-oriented assumption that people "naturally" want to do what is right.

Therefore, the 1,9-oriented nursing administrator's attitude toward mistakes and errors is "to accentuate the positive and eliminate the negative." She can do this by not blaming anyone.

"I'm sorry it happened. I know how you must feel badly about it. Perhaps if you try not to think about it and start something else, you will feel better."

The staff member is helped to find relief from any blame she may be feeling from within. The head nurse cushions a staff member in some manner such as, "Well, I know you did your best. Don't worry, things will work out." If that doesn't work, the 1,9-oriented nursing administrator is likely to coddle a troubled staff member with encouragement—all is "forgiven and forgotten."

This attitude is particularly evident when the mistake or error has been one of violating policies and procedures, particularly if unobserved by others. Under a 1,9 supervisor, orientation policies and procedures are not so rigid that people are forced to stay within them. They are guideline indicators rather than fixed or inflexible requirements. "After all, when someone is upset and confused, it is awfully difficult to walk the line." Looking at it from this angle, the 1,9-oriented nursing administrator sees no need for constant vigilance to seek out mistakes or errors. Even if a staff member does go against important policies and procedures, a nurse with a 1,9 orientation gives her no more than a gentle reminder. Another chance helps the staff nurse recognize and avoid the problem in the future, and she appreciates the nursing administrator all the more for being understanding and not getting nasty.

In the situation that follows, Marilyn, head nurse, has the intricate job of soothing feelings and keeping harmony among three people: Charles (the orderly), Ruth (staff nurse), and Dr. Gilliland.

Ruth has just obtained a urine sample from Neal Scott in Room 200. They have been running tests on Neal for two days, and Dr. Gilliland wanted to finish them by tomorrow if at all possible. Today required taking urine samples for twenty-four hours. Ruth's shift was the last remaining eight-hour period.

Ruth, with urine sample in hand, opens the door to the utility room to put the sample into Mr. Scott's urine bottle. Charles, an orderly, is standing at the sink pouring out liquid.

"Hi," says Ruth, as she goes to the shelf to get Mr. Scott's bottle.

"Hi to you," responds Charles. He empties the bottle and sets it aside to be sterilized.

"Now where in the world is it," murmurs Ruth, more to herself than anyone else. "Where's what?" asks Charles. "Mr. Scott's urine bottle. It was here yesterday." Ruth checks shelves both above and below. "Oh," says Charles. "I just poured out an unmarked bottle. I asked around and no one knew whose it was." Ruth throws her hands up in despair. "You didn't ask *me*! Dr. Gilliland is going to kill me, which is what I feel like doing to you!" She turns and stalks out, heading straight for Marilyn's desk.

Ruth explains the situation to Marilyn, who in turn comforts Ruth. "Try not to worry. I'll think of something to tell Dr. Gilliland." She knows that the urine samples will have to be started all over and that means an extra day in the hospital. She also knows that Neal Scott is counting the days when he can go home; adding one more is going to be difficult to explain. "I'll tell both Dr. Gilliland and Mr. Scott it was an unavoidable accident. After all, Charles didn't *mean* to do it. Which reminds me, I had better find Charles and tell him not to feel too badly."

This is a 1,9-oriented approach in that Marilyn's major concern was for the feelings of her staff, with little concern for the ramifications of what had happened as far as the patient is concerned, or the self-responsibility of Charles for doing his job in a proper manner. Because it is important for her to be accepted by everyone and to avoid feelings of rejection, Marilyn approached each person individually with the intention of soothing any negative feelings.

Complaints

When a 1,9-oriented nursing administrator hears complaints, these are worrisome to her, the more so if the complaints are personal. Complaints about the situation, the equipment, or the inevitable pressure are not so disturbing because she realizes that her staff does not expect her to be able to do everything. In responding to such complaints, the 1,9-oriented nursing administrator usually joins in agreeing with the complaint being expressed. This tells the staff that she is on their side. Her attitudes might be expressed in this way:

"They know I can't do anything about most complaints; therefore I try to smooth things over by telling them that I know just how they feel."

When the complaint is personal, the 1,9-oriented nursing administrator takes it at face value. When confronted with such a situation, she does everything possible to ease the feelings against her. This might involve an apology, or a promise that it will not happen again. It might mean her doing an unexpected favor—buying lunch or bringing a cake for someone's birthday. In this way, she can avoid rejection by letting staff members know that she is sorry and "Let's have no hard feelings." Such steps can take the sting out of any antagonism the staff member may have felt and replace it with a sense of harmony, even though such approaches rarely restore mutual respect.

Eleanor, a head nurse in the emergency room, yields to the pressure of complaints from her nurses and lets them take unauthorized breaks from the emergency unit to go to the nearby cafeteria for food, even though coverage of emergencies might suffer.

The emergency room staff in this particular hospital works straight eight-hour shifts with no provision for lunch break. Depending upon the casualty intake position at any given moment, a doctor, nurse, or orderly is authorized to eat outside the emergency room facilities. For this purpose a room with coffee and food-warming equipment is available a few steps away. The hospital cafeteria is considered too far away from the emergency room for personnel to be recalled with the speed required.

During one of the staff meetings, one of the registered nurses, Teri, mentions that she does not like having to bring lunch from home. Others express the same complaint. Several request permission to go to the cafeteria one at a time, with the understanding that they will hurry back as soon as called. At a fast pace, getting back takes about three minutes.

"Well, it is very unfortunate that the cafeteria isn't more conveniently near," Eleanor responds. "But we *do* have a microwave oven in the break room. Don't you find it's nice to bring food from home and warm it up there?"

"Well, some might, but with a husband and children I don't, and it's the same for others too," Teri rejoined. There were murmurs of agreement.

Eleanor is ill at ease. "Well, I'm sure that is the case. I always buy a sandwich or something in the little shop across the street before coming on duty, and I find their food quite good." Several staff members say they cannot agree. In fact, its popular name is "poison pit." Its prices are steep, and so on.

Eleanor, obviously uncomfortable, says, "Well, I suppose it would be alright if we went only for a snack in the cafeteria one at a time. Please remember to hurry back the moment you are called."

This is a 1,9-oriented response because, even though the standards are well defined by emergency room policy and procedures, Eleanor, rather than risk becoming unpopular with nurses and orderlies, surrenders and takes the most comfortable position. The impact on emergency is more or less ignored.

Hostile feelings

A 1,9-oriented nursing administrator collapses in the face of hostile feelings even more than when faced with complaints. The reason is that hostile feelings are only a few degrees removed from active dislike, and active dislike is only a step or two away from hate. For a 1,9-oriented person this path seems to lead to disaster because it gets into undermining the very foundation of that person's main security. Hostility, conflict, and antagonism are emotions that a 1,9-oriented nursing administrator does her utmost to avoid. This means that she simply wards off hostile feelings. Smoothing over these kinds of negative feelings by making believe everything is fine reduces the tensions felt even though the causes remain. The continued focus of her efforts is on trying to ensure that they are not generated at all.

A 1,9-oriented nursing administrator can attempt to reestablish harmony in many ways. The staff can be coaxed into looking at how good things are relative to how bad things might be. She may say to the staff: "Look, I know it's tough here and there are days I can't stand the place. But when I think of other units, I think we are far better off. Also, look at the job security." Her mental attitude is, "Think positively. Every cloud has a silver lining."

This kind of warm, generous acceptance toward the person who is feeling hostile, even though it does not focus on and relieve the hostility itself, can often turn the situation around, with harmony replacing the hostility previously felt. This is partly so because, when the 1,9-oriented nursing administrator reacts in a sympathetic manner, wanting to get back into a warm relationship, it is difficult for a hostile staff member to maintain her hostility. The staff member is more likely to say, "All right, let's drop it." The 1,9-oriented administrator then moves on to another topic or matter after good feelings are restored. However, not all matters that are dropped are forgotten.

Remember Marilyn, the head nurse who had to deal with the patient, Neal Scott, whose urine sample was poured down the hopper? She is still experiencing the ramifications of that situation when she arrives at home that day.

Marilyn drives her car into the driveway, turns off the engine, and just sits there for a couple of minutes. Then she slowly gets out of the car and walks into the house. Telling her husband she is exhausted, she lies down on the sofa. It seems she has been placating people all day long. Her mind drifts back to the events of the day. She can still see Ruth's face when she came out of Neal Scott's room. "That old man!" she wailed. "He told me to get out of his room. He said he had wasted enough time and expense without my causing him to stay another day. It wasn't *my* fault. Just who does he think he is? He told me Dr. Gilliland was upset about it and he's going to the director of nurses."

Marilyn tried to calm her down. "I can sympathize, Ruth. He really had no business jumping on you like that. He was rather nasty to me too. Why don't you take a break while I think of something."

The problem was that she could not think of something. She wanted to talk with Mr. Scott again but she also knew how testy he was. He liked desserts. Maybe she would call down to the kitchen and have something sent up. Maybe, just maybe, she will wake up and discover this is all just a bad dream.

This is a 1,9-oriented behavior response because Marilyn is more concerned about comforting both Ruth and Mr. Scott than in evaluating the situation for what it is and getting on with the job of providing adequate patient care.

DEVELOPMENT

Since a 1,9-oriented nursing administrator is person oriented, she is very much interested in seeing that staff members receive the necessary education to be able to perform on her unit. Orientation is to be appealing. She listens to all questions, and encourages the staff members to look up the answer. She turns it into their problem. Although not too structured, the majority of the staff are content. Her attitude is:

"I try to schedule inservice conferences and classes that will appeal to my staff. That way they can get a break from the same old routine."

Occasionally one of the staff may be a "loner," rather aloof. The 1,9-oriented nursing administrator finds this difficult to accept, perceiving it to be a personal rejection of her. She tries to figure out how to have her join the group socially. Jean, head nurse, handles this as follows.

Kay, staff nurse, has been on 3 South since this past September. She is a good registered nurse but keeps to herself. She does not usually attend outside parties and actually has little to say outside the context of work.

This aloofness worries Jean, the head nurse. She noticed not long after she hired her that Kay did not mix well with the other nurses. Jean prefers a social group and would like to know Kay better. She is concerned too that perhaps Kay does not like her.

There is a patient teaching conference in San Francisco next May, and the director of nurses has asked Jean to send someone to the conference. She is thinking about sending Kay. This would be a good opportunity to see if this might change her attitude.

By doing something that she thinks will please Kay, Jean hopes these underlying tensions will dissipate and Kay will "join" the group.

A 1,9 orientation to development is to encourage by tender loving care. A nursing administrator will treat her staff members as hothouse flowers, giving as much care and attention as is required to help growth and fulfillment to occur.

For a 1,9-oriented nursing administrator, performance evaluation can be like driving down a road that has been land-mined. The reason is her fear that any remark, no matter how well intended, may be taken by the staff member as personal criticism of her work. The staff member reacts defensively. The head nurse must either retract or defend her statement with an example.

For this reason, a 1,9-oriented nursing administrator deals very carefully in performance evaluations. Her goal is to keep things on the positive side. She is likely to operate on the proposition that people will improve by strengthening skills rather than by eliminating weaknesses. In this way, she can talk to the staff member about all the things she does well and not worry about mentioning the areas where improvement is needed.

Mary McCarthy, head nurse, approaches Betty King, staff nurse, and hands her an evaluation form, gently explaining that it needs to be signed and that since Betty is in line for a salary increase, all she has to do is put her signature on it. Betty takes the form and looks over it, saying, "But Mary, I would like to discuss some of the problems I've been faced with which has to do with some of the points contained here in the form." Mary replies, "Well, Betty, you have been here long enough to know you don't have anything to worry about. If you want to discuss it, fine, but I think you are doing a great job! Why don't you look over it and check some of the items, and if you don't agree, then I'll talk to you about them. Okay?"

This is a 1,9-oriented approach to performance evaluation. Mary has an overwhelming concern for not bringing up anything that might generate ill feelings or conflict. She prefers to avoid an evaluation discussion that might destroy the atmosphere of warmth and approval.

A 1,9-oriented administrator who seeks to change things by suggestions and innovations implies that things will be done differently. The administrator's reaction is "We're getting along so well, let's not disrupt our happy family."

INTRODUCTION OF CHANGE

Though change is inevitable, the 1,9-oriented administrative nurse full well realizes that change can be very disrupting. Therefore, change should be introduced in order to gain maximum support and minimum disruption.

A 1,9-oriented director of nurses, upon learning of the presumed advantages of the unit manager system, and seeing its potential value for solving some of the conflicts and complaints of her service, would discuss the organization shifts with the hospital director. With his approval, she would then hold a head nurse meeting, but much in advance of when the shift over to the new system would happen, and conduct it in the following manner.

"As you know, many hospitals have experimented with the unit manager system and have found that it relieves a nurse from a lot of menial paper work. A possibility that we might shift over to the unit manager system has been discussed with other people in the administration and I was thinking we might give it a try."

Before she can continue, one of the head nurses speaks up and says, "Oh no! Does that mean I would have to share my station with a lay person, probably a man, who only knows administration but knows very little or nothing about what goes on in a hospital?" Other nurses chime in, their reactions indicating that they are threatened by the possibility of being reduced in status.

The quick chorus of negative attitudes tells the 1,9-oriented director of nurses that what she thought was a good idea is likely to be anything but for her nurses.

The 1,9-oriented director of nurses would not persist but would pull back, saying, "I'm glad to see how committed all of you are to conducting your units yourself. It may very well be that the best way to proceed is to continue the way we operate now rather than try something we don't know will work well." But to avoid appearing wishy-washy at having proposed an idea and then making a 180 degree reversal, she might say, "This needs to be thought about some more, and I would like to postpone any final decision on this until we have had opportunities to interview the director of nurses in other hospitals who have adopted this plan and be sure that they can endorse it 100 percent before we decide to implement it."

In the preceding example, the 1,9-oriented director of nurses attempted to introduce what she thought would be a change that would be received positively. Upon meeting the initial resistance of her staff, she quickly pulled back. She would prefer to retract her suggestion of change rather than to meet the resistance and resentment that this possibility creates.

REACTIONS TO 1,9 SUPERVISION

Reactions to a 1,9 orientation range from feeling safe and secure within a warm and friendly atmosphere to feeling smothered and unchallenged by virtue of working in an unstimulating environment.

Security

A staff nurse or other employee who has a 1,9 orientation finds her desire for approval reinforced and her fear of rejection unfounded. The 1,9-oriented administrative atmosphere is supportive and helpful. When asked about her attitudes, a staff member under a 1,9-oriented nursing administrator says, "I would not want to change jobs. I enjoy the people I work with. I couldn't ask for better conditions of comfort and security."

The head nurse remarks, "Several units here have high turnover but not mine. Most of my girls have been here for years. That's because we have a low-key atmosphere rather than a pressure cooker. We all like one another, we work well together, everything is positive."

Similarly, a 1,9-oriented director of nursing might say, "My nursing staff is very content. We have no real turnover. In comparison with the hospital across town, we have wonderful morale. As a matter of fact, we have a waiting list of people who want to come to work for us."

Resentment and frustration

The reactions just cited are not universal. They are limited to those whose orientations are 1,9 in character. A nurse with a 9,1 orientation would find it too stifling and unstructured. Suggestions for change go unheeded. Many staff nurses find challenging work rewarding, with stimulation originating in the work itself. When such people are not challenged, frustration arises because, even though they may be paid well, they may feel that they are wasting time and making little or no contribution. By failing to endorse open communication and resolve conflicts, whether it is between doctor, aides, or hospital administration, a 1,9-oriented nursing administrator may provoke frustrations that she most devoutly seeks to avoid.

SUMMARY

The 1,9-oriented style of supervision emphasizes the overriding importance of good relations. The theory is that, if staff members are happy, contented, and feel a sense of warmth, self-worth, and acceptance, they then want to cooperate.

The director of nurses, the head nurse, or other supervisor is always in the middle between two layers, and how she acts to link these layers is an important aspect of her administration. The 1,9-oriented administrative nurse does this by trying to please everyone, whether a layer above or her staff nurses, though her first loyalty lies with the nurses in her unit.

Planning and scheduling, execution, and follow-up all share in common an underlying dynamic when 1,9-oriented supervision is involved. The 1,9-oriented nurse's efforts to give general rather than close supervision are based on the premise that staff nurses will give more support to a general kind of supervision than when being told precisely what to do.

A second aspect of her administration is concerned with delegation. The 1,9-oriented administrative nurse makes use of delegation because, by doing so, she reduces or eliminates potential disagreements between herself and those who are expected to carry something out. She, in turn, can take whatever the staff nurse does under a policy of delegation and give it her maximum support and encouragement.

Communications are seen as at the very heart of good relationships. Any topic that provides an opportunity for people to share their thoughts and feelings and emotions in a mutually appreciative way is okay. Directions are offered in a general fashion, always with the anticipation and hope that staff members will be asking questions. And as they do, they will begin to feel "ownership" of the problem or issue, making close supervision unnecessary.

Mistakes and errors are best dealt with by not tackling them head on. The better approach under these conditions is to give subordinates forgiveness reinforced with understanding and support.

Complaints are likely to be dealt with by the head nurse agreeing that the situation is unfortunate or just too bad and trying to shift attention away by getting staff members to agree that "every cloud has a silver lining," or in some other way to smooth over the difference and to get people to be nice to one another. When hostile feelings are expressed, the nursing administrator apologizes, if that is appropriate, or makes amends, if that will help restore good relations.

Development is best accomplished with the assumption that staff members are helped to progress more by emphasizing their strengths and by assisting them to improve what they already do well, rather than by harping on deficiencies that they can do very little about correcting anyway. Thus a 1,9-oriented nursing administrator conducts performance evaluation in a manner that causes subordinates to feel complimented rather than criticized.

Changes are introduced, and the 1,9-oriented nursing administrator is always taken aback when a proposal or a request or a suggestion is questioned or challenged. She does not persist and thereby create win-lose positions, but rather capitulates, if that is possible; if it is not, she draws back the proposal of change in some such way that allows "further study," with the longer-term prospect that the proposed change will never reappear for consideration.

Chapter 5

THE 1,1-ORIENTED NURSING ADMINISTRATOR

Although she has emotionally resigned and retreated into indifference, the 1,1-oriented nursing administrator's motivation is to remain in her job. This means doing enough to preserve her job without making much of an effort to contribute to the benefit of her colleagues or the hospital agency. She expects little and gives little in return. Although she may appear bored, drifting, and listless, if this does not expose her to expulsion, she is prepared to put up with the situation as she goes through the rituals of being a nurse in charge.

On the negative side, her motivation is to hold on and avoid sinking into hopelessness and despair or being dismissed. By being visible yet inconspicuous, she escapes being controversial, having enemies, or getting fired. She is likely to appear somewhat preoccupied, and these attitudes keep others off her back. The degree to which she remains tacit, unresponsive, and uninvolved is governed by the acceptable minimum others are prepared to tolerate. By not becoming emotionally entangled with tasks or people, she avoids coming to grips with her inadequacies and inabilities. This combination of neutrality and physical presence is the key to being able to keep from provoking undue resentment by others because of her noncommitment. Her motto is, "See no evil, speak no evil, hear no evil, and you are protected by not being noticed."

How is it possible for a hospital to ignore its deadwood? It is well known that in many hospitals a nursing administrator is rarely fired; if she has been in her position for any length of time, it is her job until retirement. A better question might be, "How does a 1,1-oriented nursing administrator get promoted into the position of head nurse or director of nurses?" She might be promoted simply because of seniority; or she may have been a good technician, and this is what led to her advancement, regardless of the fact that she may have lacked leadership and administrative abilities. Or, there was a need for a person in this position and she was available.

Characteristics of the 1,1-oriented nursing administrator are apparent in various ways. She is neither warm nor cold nor responsive nor negative. Then how can she be described? Bland, opaque, plastic. You might think of one of those store-window figures, wired for sound and transferred to your organization, and yet you know that she must somehow be alive because she breathes and moves, arrives and leaves, and, in between, eats.

A 1,1-oriented nursing administrator, however, may not have always been passive and indifferent. She may have been involved and somewhere along the way she may have been "burned." She tried to help the staff, the patients, and got hurt or defeated in a clash of personalities and vowed that she would never get involved or become concerned again over what happens at work. Possibly patients for whom she had developed affection died. Perhaps accidents happened to patients that were too traumatic for her to deal with emotionally. Gradually she withdrew, preferring to administer her duties only in a technical fashion and creating barriers that served as protective walls for her total being.

Another possibility is that, after years of performing well in an administrative capacity, the position is no longer challenging. She feels drained and is burned out. Her private rationalization may be that she wishes to spend more time with family and friends. She may even rationalize her 1,1 attitudes and escape her situation by study at a nearby school. Sometimes withdrawal into a 1,1 orientation results when she no longer can fight back and yet cannot afford to leave to seek employment elsewhere.

A 1,1-oriented nurse rationalizes her lack of participation by placing the blame on someone or something else. An example is, "Hospitals have become so big that nothing can be done about it. They have become very dehumanized and seem to be more concerned about technology. I'm putting in my eight hours but I really don't want anything to do with it any longer." She may even complain about her educational program failing to prepare her to take care of the responsibilities on a unit. These rationalizations serve the purpose of justifying indifference, passivity, and a "Who cares?" attitude, which make it unnecessary for her to have to admit to herself that she is no longer mentally and emotionally involved. As long as others leave her alone and pick up the slack, she is content to treadmill through her employment, an onlooker to her own professional career.

NURSE IN THE MIDDLE

As with any nursing administrator, the 1,1-oriented nursing administrator is faced with inevitable pressure, dissatisfactions, and unhappy or resentful staff members. Staff members have certain expectations from the nurse in charge. One of them is that she will represent or "fight" for them on their behalf. The 1,1-oriented nursing administrator usually does not take sides between those above her and those below, preferring to remain neutral in order to be noncontroversial. She becomes very adept at responding to either level without presenting any personal points of view. When asked what other people think or would do, she responds with a variety of neutral answers: "I don't know." "I haven't heard." "I wasn't on duty when it happened." "I haven't read that memo." "I never received it." When pressed further, she provides equally adept answers: "It's up to you." "Whatever you say; you're the expert."

Interactions between doctors and the director of nurses provide the perfect opportunity for buck passing. To the director of nurses she reports, ". . . it's the doctor's fault or responsibility." To the doctor, ". . . it's the director of nurses or the staff." In the following example, we see how Lillian Grant, director of nurses, reacts to years of working between various levels in the hospital structure.

Lillian Grant has been director of nurses at Plane Medical Center for twelve years, having been promoted after many years as head nurse on 4 East. The last two years have been unusually rough ones for her, as the hospital has undergone rapid expansion mainly because two large industrial companies moved into the city. The hospital has added one new ward of twenty-two beds and construction is under way for a complete wing to be completed by the end of the year. Lillian has had the responsibility of hiring four nurses plus coping with additional budgetary requirements and training programs. These increased responsibilities have resulted in Lillian looking forward to retirement. She finds it difficult to be enthusiastic about her position or the interfaces she must maintain with others during working hours.

The relationship with the chairman of the board of trustees is the least to be desired. Dr. V. O. Giles has been in that position only six months. He is precise, authoritative, and a stickler for detail. Although Lillian goes out of her way to avoid contact with him, she is always cordial in any face-to-face circumstance.

Lillian is now sitting at her desk, idly looking through the stacks of forms—interview forms, registration forms, evaluation forms. Her eyes move to the memo just received from Dr. Giles on a new suggested method of teaching patient care, with a personalized note on the bottom that she and Vincent Guard, the hospital administrator, might give strong consideration to adopting this new method at Plane Medical Center.

She lays the memo aside; she will give it thought tomorrow. She then stuffs the forms into a file folder with a silent promise to herself that she will give them to Sue, one of the administrative secretaries, to complete. Sue seems to enjoy doing the duties Lillian has delegated to her over the past year.

The intercom buzzes, jolting Lillian out of her thoughts. "Lillian? This is Vincent. I have just been told that Harrison Caldwell has been admitted to the hospital. As a big contributor to the new wing you know he deserves the suite on 2 West. Joan says it's taken."

"If it's already taken, I really don't know what can be done, Vincent. It's taken." Lillian glances at her watch. Only five minutes until quitting time; she doesn't need a problem now.

"Well, for one thing, get the administrative office to switch with whoever is in there—do something! That guy pitched in $50,000!" The phone clicks. Taking a deep breath Lillian dials the administrative office and hears the familiar voice of Joan, the administrative nurse. "I know," Joan says, "you don't have to tell me. I've already heard, Lillian. But how can I ask Mr. Gordon to move? We *promised* him that suite for his entire stay."

Lillian tries to muster some sympathy as she says, "I understand, but you've already got the word. Don't worry about it. Do whatever seems best. If Mr. Caldwell is hurting bad enough, he won't care where he's put." Lillian's watch says five minutes after five as she puts down the receiver. "Oh, no," she thinks, "I'm going to hit the traffic jam *again!*"

As the nurse in the middle, she takes no stand, letting others take initiative and responsibility as they will. Lillian, for a combination of reasons, is "burned out." Her primary concern at this point is "getting out," and the effect of this is felt not only by the administrative nurse but also by her staff and the patients as well. Others adjust to this reality, and soon accept it as a "given," and come to expect no more from her.

ADMINISTRATIVE ASPECTS OF NURSING

The production requirements of patient care are revealed in the nurse's attitudes toward planning and scheduling, execution, and follow-up.

Planning and scheduling

A 1,1-oriented nursing administrator assigns staff members to whatever tasks must be done and gives them more or less full discretion in completing them. She leaves them alone, letting them do their work, good or bad, as they see fit. She has this attitude about planning and scheduling:

"I give broad assignments and do the necessary scheduling; otherwise, though, I don't think in terms of goals or objectives. The staff fairly well supervise themselves."

Rationalizing this abdication as delegation, the nurse avoids interfering, not because others need the opportunity to be autonomous and to learn from their own efforts, but out of her own lack of involvement. The key word is delegate. After all, she has certain authority and a full staff for delegation purposes.

As the nurse in charge, she gives the impression of always being busy, of always being at her desk, and of maintaining a good attendance record. The "goal" of being busy at her desk is to be seen but unnoticed so that she is not labeled as a troublemaker, or a slacker for that matter. The deeper reason for being busy is that staff nurses will not likely interrupt her. This allows her to avoid making any decision. The goal of her "business" is to coast along until retirement.

The following example reveals how a 1,1-oriented nursing administrator, Ellie, carries out her role in planning the activities on any given day.

Ellie, head nurse, is sitting at her desk this morning, going over the assignments for the day. She sees a note she wrote yesterday reminding her that a group of student nurses are coming today. Ellie groans. She hates the interference and she has already forgotten to tell the staff they are coming. "Oh, well, no big deal," she thinks. "They only come once a month, stay two days, and then we don't see them again. Somebody will see them and will offer to change off assignments. We'll just wait 'til they get here." She yawns and stretches, wishing the day were over. She has a lot of things to do at home.

"But," she reminds herself, "another day, another dollar."

Ellie has quit taking her responsibilities for planning seriously, even on a short-term basis, assuming that things will eventually fall into place. There is likelihood in this particular situation that not only will the rest of the staff be irritated at this planning by default, but also the expectations of the students and their clinical instructor will be violated. But she also knows that once the crisis, created by failure to anticipate through planning, is over, all will be forgotten. Next year the clinical instructor will say, "Let's not go back to that unit." Now, as she prefers, Ellie is truly left alone.

Execution

Once assignments and scheduling are made, the matter of doing the activities is left entirely to the staff. Rationalizing that her staff members are professional nurses and know what they are doing, the 1,1-oriented nurse does not keep up with what they are doing, not because she thinks the staff needs to be autonomous and learn from their own experience, but because of her own lack of involvement.

"Since they know their own jobs and capabilities better than anyone else, the staff carries out their assignments as best they can."

Sylvia Carlson is a patient and her transfer is one that normally would be carried out with no problem. But because of the low involvement of Kathleen, head nurse, it turns out to be more of a trial-and-error process.

It is Sylvia Carlson's twentieth day in the hospital, having had a leg amputated, which resulted in complications. Leah, the new day nurse, has told her that today she will be moved to a semiprivate room down the hall since she has recuperated well enough to share a room with someone and the private room she is in is needed for another patient. Sylvia agrees to all this and is waiting for Leah to come in during morning rounds.

Meanwhile, Leah and Kathleen, head nurse, are discussing assignments and the prospect of moving Sylvia. "Good luck," says Kathleen, as she busies herself with paperwork, "she has enough plants in her room to open a flower shop."

Shortly thereafter Leah has an emergency with a patient and finds herself running behind schedule. Kathleen seems to be nowhere around. Finally, about eleven o'clock, Leah goes into Sylvia's room and begins transferring the gifts and plants. "Oh my, I didn't realize you had accumulated so many!" Sylvia remains silent, visibly perturbed at having to wait. She had expected Leah much earlier and the positive anticipation she had had of moving was beginning to wear off.

It takes Leah a good while to move Sylvia's things, and she stops at one point to get an orderly to help. Again, Kathleen is never seen.

Later, word comes to Kathleen that the moving process did not go well.

Kathleen's 1,1 approach was to keep out of the action by appearing to be busy or out of sight. She had no intention of seeing that Leah's assignment was carried out. As a result, Leah is not properly supervised and the care for Ms. Carlson is slipshod, coming close to creating a new problem.

Follow-up

The 1,1-oriented nurse does little by way of follow-up. She takes minimum responsibility in seeing that something has been done, and even what little follow-up she performs is done in a superficial way. Mentally she has walked out of the hospital; the less effort required to function in her role, the better.

"I make rounds and in this way I let patients know I'm in charge, but I take little on-the-spot action if I can avoid it. The staff likes it that way; I do, too."

There are occasions, however, when it is necessary to follow up on a particular situation, but it is usually because it is demanded, either directly by the doctor, her immediate superior, a patient, or a crisis of circumstances in the situation itself.

Remember the episode in Chapter 4 about drawing blood? Let's do an "instant replay" and see how Martha, head nurse, would have reacted had she been dealing with the problem from a 1,1 orientation.

Jennifer, staff nurse, is beginning to lose her patience. She cannot locate a vein in the arm of the patient, Paul Burn. She has tried twice and now Mr. Burn is beginning to show his uneasiness. On Jennifer's third attempt, he asks exasperatingly, "Would you get someone who knows how to take blood!" Jennifer hastily leaves the room, saying, "I'll be back in a minute." She leaves the room and approaches Martha at the nurse's station. "I can't get blood from Mr. Burn this morning. I tried three times."

"Really? Well, why don't you see if Grace can do it. I think she's in 201 right now. Anyway, that's where she said she was going a minute ago." She returns to her order book.

We see that Martha makes no effort to help Jennifer to learn to draw properly nor did she indicate any real concern for Mr. Burn. Instead, she referred Jennifer to another person for assistance, thereby relieving herself of the responsibility of follow-up teaching of one of her staff.

COMMUNICATION

There are a number of ways in which a 1,1-oriented nursing administrator goes about communicating with her staff and others. In terms of giving directions, she will often say, "Here is what is to be done. Let me know when you're finished." Then she leaves staff members alone, letting them do their work as they see fit, and hoping they will solve their problems by getting help from one another rather than coming back for assistance. For example, she is not likely to ask questions because they might provoke additional concerns with which she then would have to deal. She prefers to leave it up to the staff to ask questions on the assumption that each staff member is supposed to know what she needs to know. In thinking about a staff member, the 1,1-oriented nurse says to herself, "If she wants the information, she'll ask for it." If she does, the administrative nurse answers it if she knows, and she promises to find out if she does not.

More than likely someone on her staff is the surrogate nursing administrator, as anyone who works under the 1,1 orientation soon learns that there is little give and take in the sense of real communication. When the staff nurses learn to rely on one another, the 1,1-oriented head nurse compliments herself on promoting "teamwork."

When it comes to listening, a 1,1-oriented nurse is not too attentive nor is she emotionally involved with staff members' problems. She prefers to let them talk with one another as she tunes herself out and thinks about other things— shopping lists, needlepoint, the menu for dinner, and so on. If a remark is made or a question repeated, she can always say, "I'm sorry. I didn't get what you said." A result of this kind of attitude is that others mistakenly consider her thoughtful and one who does not make impulsive comments. Her silence may even come through to others as profound.

When it comes to implementing necessary communications, the 1,1-oriented nursing administrator is a message carrier. At meetings with her colleagues, she takes note after note, which gives the impression that she is very much involved. This also gives her a record of what has been going on. She dutifully carries orders down the line from above, repeating the message exactly as she heard it. When she meets with her staff to keep them informed, she reads all of her notes to them. There are no questions. If anyone does ask one, her comment can be, "They didn't talk about it." Thereafter, if anything goes wrong, it is because they didn't listen. She can report back, and correctly, that she "told" them and they didn't listen.

How a 1,1-oriented nursing administrator passes down information is shown in the following example. Carleen, head nurse, makes even less effort to get a question answered by one of her staff.

Carleen is reading a memo she received this morning from Fran Nolan, director of nurses, regarding staff attendance at in-service meetings. Ms. Nolan wants to know why Carleen's unit has had the lowest attendance record. Carleen considers putting it in her "hold" folder. Those meetings are just a waste of time anyway. If the staff doesn't want to go she isn't going to push them. They can make up their own minds. But since she has some other items to pass along to the staff from the director, she may as well read this one at the meeting this afternoon too.

The meeting is convened that afternoon and Carleen reads the memo about the in-service meetings.

"Carleen, do we *have* to go?" asks Sue, a staff nurse.

"That's what it says. Policy stipulates that a staff nurse should not miss more than two a year," responds Carleen.

"But sometimes I just don't have the time," objects Sue. "Could you check and see if we have any alternative?"

"Well, I'll think about it and see what I can do. I'll talk to Ms. Nolan about it when I get a chance." Carleen lays the memo aside.

Several days later Sue meets Ms. Nolan in the hallway and asks whether she has made a decision on the requirement to attend the in-service meeting.

"Well, actually I didn't know you had any objections," says a surprised Ms. Nolan. "Carleen never mentioned it."

Carleen used a 1,1-oriented approach to communication. She failed to respond to Sue's request and probably has no intention of doing so. It will not take more than a couple of incidences similar to this one before staff members will realize that Carleen cannot be depended upon to take a straightforward approach in letting the director of nurses know their feelings. In this situation, most likely she will simply ignore policy until someone pressures her to comply.

In the following example, Lisa, staff nurse, finds herself becoming frustrated at Cora, the head nurse, who has not told her about a change in procedure that can affect her personally.

Lisa, staff nurse, steps off the elevator and approaches Cora, head nurse, who is sitting at the nurse's station filing her nails.

"Cora, I just heard there's a new procedure on picking up paychecks at Payroll."

"Really?" Cora asks more or less disinterestedly as she laboriously works at a hangnail.

"Yes, in fact, Jane, the nurse on 6 West, just told me. Did you know?" Lisa could feel herself getting more and more irritated. Trying to get something out of Cora is like pulling teeth.

Cora puts down her file. "Well, now that you mention it, there is a memo floating around here somewhere. In fact, I think we talked about it in our last meeting."

"That was the day I had to leave early," Lisa replies.

Cora shrugs her shoulders and picks up her file and starts filing her nails on the other hand. "Oh, well, why worry about it. You'll get your check one way or another."

Lisa's irritation at Cora's lack of involvement is hardly contained. Cora had quit worrying about such details long ago. And why get all bothered? After all, she had done what she was supposed to. It wasn't her fault Lisa missed the meeting.

CONFLICT

The best way to handle conflict is to avoid it. But how does a nursing administrator do it? First, she keeps up the appearance of being busy. It does not make any difference what she does, as long as she is occupied. There may be papers all over her desk; she may have papers in her hand as she walks down the corridor. If she looks busy, often the staff will feel guilty were they to interrupt her.

When confronted in a potential conflict situation, the 1,1-oriented nurse reacts by remaining neutral, or she may withdraw from the situation entirely. The way to deal with a memo she does not like is to delay in responding to it, discard or file it, and immediately forget all about it. She can always say, "I didn't get it."

Another way to manage conflict is to delay confronting it by accepting the problem and then pretending to study the situation. She knows that if she delays long enough, the problem will likely go away. The resolution always slips into the future. If the problem lingers, she lets someone higher up take over.

Mistakes and errors

A 1,1-oriented nursing administrator overlooks mistakes and errors by ignoring them when this can be done without her being confronted. The only time she may take action is if she knows that persons higher up will find out and she herself will be called on the carpet. To avoid as much conflict as possible she places responsibility in such a way as to be relieved from being accountable; the strategy is to delegate responsibility to others without appearing to pass the buck.

The 1,1-oriented nurse usually has excuses that serve as self-protectors so that accusation or blame can be avoided. Her attitude is that mistakes are more or less inevitable: "Since you can't do much about them, why worry?"

In the following example, Joyce, a charge nurse, shifts the blame rather than making sure that the LPN, Norma, is properly trained.

Dr. Neely has finished rounds and approaches Joyce at the nurse's station. He says, "Mrs. Cook didn't get the treatment to her back that I ordered."

Joyce looks up from her reading. "I'll check on it, but it was probably the new LPN," she says. As she leaves the nurse's station, she meets the new LPN, Norma. "Dr. Neely tells me you didn't give Mrs. Cook her back treatment; she was supposed to have one around ten o'clock."

"But I didn't know it was ordered," responds Norma.

Joyce shrugs and says, "The doctor wrote the order after he finished rounds. It's in the order book."

"I have been very busy, and I couldn't get to the desk to check," Norma replies. "At the last hospital I worked in, if a new order was written, the charge nurse came and told me."

"I normally don't," says Joyce. "Every staff has her own responsibilities to keep abreast of the order book. You had better write it up on the incident report. I don't want to be blamed for it later."

Joyce makes sure that she is not held responsible for any errors. She puts the blame back on the staff nurse, assuaging her conscience by, "After all, I do give them freedom. They must learn to assume more responsibility." Mistakes and errors, then, tend to persist and repeat themselves unless they are caught, often accidentally, by someone else. When this happens it is often found that the 1,1-oriented nurse who should be responsible has shifted the blame and passed the responsibility onward to someone else.

Complaints

The 1,1-oriented nursing administrator seeks to steer her relationships with her subordinates along a complaint-free path. She avoids being open to subordinates' complaints, and yet the staff cannot describe her as ignoring them either. The easiest way to avoid getting involved is not to get drawn into someone else's problems. Once a complaint is raised, the strategy is to acknowledge it with a brief "Hmm, that's bad" type of comment to imply giving further thought. Then, for all practical purposes, it is forgotten. Or the response may be, "Yes, I know. That's one of the big hang-ups around here. But they soon see you as a troublemaker if you try to do anything about it." The implication is to go along with it, for whatever it is worth. Neutrality makes it possible to live in a world where one sees no disagreement. Her basic attitude can be summed up in this way.

"Why get stirred up when someone complains? There will always be someone with problems. Me? I just let them go in one ear and out the other."

Sometimes a staff nurse may try to get a 1,1-oriented supervisor to do something specific about a complaint. She persists even after being told, "Sorry, but that is something I can't do anything about." For example, a staff member begins to talk about going up through channels, and the head nurse may begin to feel a little uncomfortable. She may shift the conversation by indicating a readiness to consult the next level in the organization to get the answer. After a period of time has elapsed, the subordinate wants to know what has happened. The head nurse is likely to respond with, "There doesn't seem to be a policy on that" or "They couldn't decide, so I guess they're going to take it further upstairs."

If the staff member continues to press the complaint and asks for help on what to do next, the 1,1-oriented head nurse is likely to say, "It's up to you" or

"I wouldn't want to influence your decision" or "You might want to go see so-and-so." "There are all kinds of pros and cons, and I'm not an expert on it." Another typical 1,1-oriented response is, "Well, there are two ways you might go about it, but you probably will have a better feel than I for which is best."

Gwin, a head nurse, is faced with the prospect of getting authorization to add a utility room as a result of a complaint from Celia, a staff nurse. Gwin brushes the remark aside by saying, "I can't do anything about it." In this way she fails to respond adequately to the complaint or to ease the situation in any way.

Celia has finally reached the point of impatience because all of the equipment she needs to work with is kept in the utility room in the other wing. Even though she has tried to anticipate her needs, she always seems to run out or need something different. This necessitates taking time away from patient care. Today she decides to complain to Gwin, the head nurse.

"Gwin," Celia begins, "I'm tired of having to go get supplies. Can't we set up a small supply closet in this wing so we won't have to be away from our patients so long? It takes us so much longer to complete our assignments!"

"I'm afraid I can't do anything about it. That would be a big project."

"Not really. Portable shelves would do," Celia replies. "We have to do something. Sometimes I run myself ragged."

"I'll think about it; maybe I'll talk to the supervisor about it, but you know how tight money is right now," responds Gwin.

Time passes. A month later Celia is still having to go to the other wing for supplies. One day she sees the unit supervisor and teases her about how long it is taking for the shelves to come in. Of course she finds out that Gwin never mentioned them, much less ordered them.

Hostile feelings

A 1,1-oriented nursing administrator reacts to hostile feelings by keeping her cool since she has no intention of being drawn in. Getting a polite or poker-faced reaction or no reply at all, the staff members are likely to say, either aloud or to themselves, "You can't get blood from a turnip, so to heck with it," and walk away.

A 1,1-oriented administrative nurse wears down her subordinates' hostile feelings in much the same way that a skillful angler plays a fish until it is played out. She may listen silently. Whenever the staff member ceases, she waits. She might even be skillful enough to act as if she is about to interrupt the subordinate, but quickly yields the floor when the subordinate starts up again. In this way, she prompts the staff member time and time again to vent her anger until eventually the staff member has nothing more to say and no harm has been done. Indeed the ventilation may itself have a cathartic effect, which takes the frustration out of the problem. They might even walk away together. The nursing administrator's attitude might be as follows.

"I can't help it if people get upset. I've learned to just let it bounce off. It often helps them to feel better if I let them complain."

It is easier to describe a 1,1-oriented nursing administrator's way of reacting to hostile feelings by describing what it is *not*. She does not actively seek to become aware of hostile feelings that may have been brought about by the character of her supervision, but neither does she make an effort to run away from them. In a certain sense the 1,1-oriented nurse accepts the expressions of hostile feelings like the walls of a soundproof room. While the staff nurse does not get punished or criticized, she knows deep down that having made the effort made her feel better even though it did not change much. The same old situation will be around tomorrow, the next day, and next year.

A 1,1-oriented approach to dealing with hostile feelings is evident in the following situation. Gladys, head nurse, does not even consider the staff nurses' feelings important enough to warrant any real discussion.

Nothing seems to be going right for Lenora, staff nurse on 2 West. She woke up late and had trouble starting the car. There was no parking available when she came in so, when she came on duty, she was angry and frustrated, only to find that beginning next Monday she is assigned to 3 West for two weeks because they are shorthanded. All the nurses are upset about it. There are distinct ill feelings between the two units. The subject comes up while they are charting.

Addressing Gladys, the head nurse, Lenora says, "Gladys, I just don't understand why we have to help out on 3 West. Whenever we need someone, you can just bet they won't come up here. They think surgical unit is the pits."

Gladys sits back and listens. Several of the other nurses pick up on Lenora's remarks, indicating that no one has a good thing to say about their unit except when they need help. Margaret, who has been on the same unit with Gladys for five years, mutters loud enough for all to hear, "Maybe they have a point." Finally, Gladys says, "Oh, don't worry about it, don't pay any attention to them; it's just the way they are. They've got to complain about something." She gets up and glances at her watch, which signals that the break is over and it's time to go back to work.

This is a 1,1-oriented reaction because Gladys clearly adopted a "do nothing" attitude and offered no constructive comments, much less proposing anything about getting better rapport between her unit and 3 West. The assumption is that these feelings are par for the course and that if they are ignored they eventually will disappear.

DEVELOPMENT

When it comes to bringing aboard a new staff member, the 1,1-oriented nursing administrator gives the person free rein to explore, visit whom she wishes, and become acquainted in her own way. The extreme of it is, "Come back when you are through." This method of initiating new staff is acceptable if the new member knows what to look for. If it is a recent graduate nurse, with little or no idea of what it is that one needs to find out, the new nurse is up against it. She will flounder, relying on trial and error to learn what she needs to know.

Planned development is practically nonexistent in the 1,1-oriented nurse's thinking. She will send the quotas to the mandatory programs even though many times the staff may go on their own. She neither encourages nor discourages the staff. If she is told to go to a program, she herself goes without fighting it. It is as good to be in a course as on the unit. It even breaks the boredom to go once in awhile.

Generally the 1,1-oriented nurse feels that development should be initiated by the individual.

"The opportunities are there. If they (the staff) are interested, it's their choice."

Cheryl is a recent graduate nurse who is having an orientation interview with the head nurse, Lanell, before actually beginning employment on 3 West.

"Since you've been to the in-service department, Cheryl," Lanell begins, "I assume you know all about vacation time, pay schedule, and so on. Do you have any questions about that?"

"No," replied Cheryl. "I may later but I think I have all the essential information. I am a little nervous, though. This is my first full-time job."

"You'll soon get over that," says Lanell. "In fact, it won't be long before you'll wish you were back in school! It gets dull pretty quick!" She glances at her watch and continues, "I don't have anything further. When you come in Monday, I'll put you with somebody—I don't know who yet. Almost anyone around here can help if you have any questions or problems."

Taking that to mean the end of the meeting, Cheryl gets up to leave. "Will see you Monday," Lanell says, and turns her attention to tidying her desk.

Lanell's 1,1-oriented approach is evident in the more-or-less disinterested manner in which she orients Cheryl to her role as a staff member. She makes no effort to investigate Cheryl's goals or what kind of practice experience she has had. To Lanell, she is just someone to fill a gap.

The 1,1-oriented nursing administrator carries out performance evaluation as a matter of policy. She fills out whatever forms are required by the agency, but little thought goes into the writing. To do otherwise brings unwanted attention and queries from above. If the hospital policy requires that she have a conference with each of the staff members, she does so. The individual is given a mechanical explanation, asked if there are any questions, and then asked to sign in the proper space. The interview is complete.

In the following example, Nita, head nurse, administers her evaluation of Renee in a perfunctory manner. She fills in "satisfactory" and considers the matter finished.

Renee, a staff nurse, is approached in the hall by Nita, the head nurse, who says, "Renee, after you're through with Mrs. Elkins' bath, check with me on your evaluation report."

Later Renee joins Nita at the nurses' station. "I've gone over the sheet, Renee. You've been here a year and I think you've performed satisfactorily. I've checked everything that way so, if you agree, all you do is sign the sheet."

"But, Nita, I really have been pushing hard this last six months. Is that all I get— 'satisfactory'? I really need a merit raise; the money is important to me right now."

"I think as long as you fall in the 'satisfactory' column, that's all you have to worry about," Nita replies. "You shouldn't have any problem with that. Oh, there goes Mr. Lyon's buzzer. You had better check with him. If you want to talk further about a raise you can see the director of nurses."

This is a 1,1-oriented approach because Nita obviously takes little interest in whether the evaluation is an objective appraisal of Renee's performance or of the feelings she has about the rating.

INTRODUCTION OF CHANGE

Innovation is not a 1,1-oriented nursing administrator's strong suit. As a matter of fact, the introduction of change takes energy, and a nurse with this orientation has a short supply of it. Yet changes are inevitable and even a 1,1-oriented director of nurses is asked to make changes in her service by those above her.

Her way of dealing with such requests is to take them almost in literal form. She makes the request in the form that she receives it, adding no further information from her own resourcefulness. If staff nurses resist, she says, "They said they wanted it that way, and I suspect that that's what we'll have to do." Her manner of dealing with the expected change conveys no enthusiasm, and she gives no emotional support. Yet she is not subject to criticism if failure results, because she had let it be known to the staff that the change had been imposed upon her.

A director of nurses, Carolyn, receives a call from the hospital administrator, Bill, who says, "I would like to sit down with you and review the unit manager plan. I think a number of your problems could be solved by getting someone to help in this capacity. Could you meet at 1:15?" Carolyn replies, "Of course."

At 1:15 Carolyn meets with Bill, who explains the unit manager role. She listens, without responding one way or another, except to say at one point that it might be worth a try. He says, "We think that this is a good idea, but before we decide upon it we would like to have the reactions of your staff. Why don't you talk it over with them and see if they have any ideas."

Carolyn says, "Okay, I'll tell them about this and let you know their reactions." Later she calls a meeting of her staff and says, "Bill told me that they are considering the unit manager plan. He wanted me to make this known to you, and to come back with whatever reactions you might have. What are your reactions?"

In the example above we see a 1,1-oriented director of nurses carrying a message from one level to another with no embroidery, no editing, no support, no recommendation. Simultaneously, though, it should be noticed that she does not disparage the idea, she does not denounce it, nor does she discourage her staff nurses from giving open consideration to the plan.

This example affords a good illustration of how a 1,1-oriented director of nurses can stay in the saddle for an extended period of time, and yet really contribute nothing to the hospital effort. As a message passer, she is on her toes, because to fail to pass along the message would subject her to criticism. In doing so, however, she avoids anything but nominal participation in the issues involved, and in this way avoids the pressures or tensions or conflicts with which she would otherwise have to deal.

REACTIONS TO 1,1 SUPERVISION

The day-to-day aspects and effects from 1,1-oriented nurse supervision have been presented. We now need to understand the longer-term implications of this approach.

Leaving

A common response to being managed in a 1,1 way is to recognize the situation for what it is, which does not mean that it is acceptable. A staff member may find herself offended by this kind of leadership and rather than adjust to it, recognize its dead-end qualities and ask for a transfer or leave.

Going all out

The staff nurse who is eager for leg room may find a 1,1-oriented nursing administrator ideal. If the individual is self-initiating, she does not even notice the absence of her supervisor. She is happy in her work and misinterprets the supervisor's abdication as delegation and this she interprets as approval of her competency. She soon may notice that the unit runs well despite the absence of supervision. After a while, however, she may also come to recognize the fact that if she really wants something, she has to bypass the nursing administrator and go directly to someone higher up.

Into 1,1

A third response to 1,1-oriented leadership is for staff nurses themselves to accept the circumstances as inevitable and to move into the 1,1 corner, receiving a paycheck in exchange for the monotony and boredom of it all. This is most likely, though, when a staff member already is headed in a 1,1 direction, and the movement is completed by transferring her from a current assignment where she may not be doing well into a setting with a 1,1-oriented supervisor who will not complain. This movement of people is said to be made necessary because "We can't sacrifice production, but we can't discharge unproductive people either. What are you going to do?" Tolerance for such 1,1 attitudes is built into many organizations, accepting the situation with futility, particularly where bureaucratic regulations or union constraints prohibit or severely limit firing. After all, every nurse is a pair of hands.

SUMMARY

A 1,1-oriented nursing administrator does the minimum of what is required until she reaches retirement. The goal is to convert a salary into a pension. The name of the game is "take it easy." She develops the skill of being visible and looking occupied without actually being seen or being productive. She contributes as little as possible without getting into trouble. The basic approach can be summarized in the following way.

Planning and scheduling, execution, and follow-up are all terms that convey the notion that something is being managed in a thoughtful way. By comparison, 1,1-oriented nursing supervision is a stimulus-response environment. This means that little or no thought is given to planning and scheduling beyond the minimum, that staff members are left on their own to instruct themselves, and that follow-up is absent except when pressure is applied from above.

Communication tends to consist of passing down and reporting upward whatever information the next higher level requests.

Staff members are left on their own initiative to determine the best way to carry out whatever assignments they have been given. Mistakes and errors are inevitable and the way *not* to get in trouble about them is to not see them.

The way a 1,1-oriented nursing administrator deals with the staff may or may not cause them to complain. She does not go around hunting for complaints, yet she does "listen" when complaints are expressed. This "listening" is done in a special way. The likelihood is that after a period of time the person doing the complaining drops it anyway.

When reacting to hostile feelings, a 1,1-oriented nursing administrator does not try to avoid them by escaping from the situation or by hiding, but neither does she feel personally involved. The attitude is that, if you do not react, pretty soon the person with the hostile feelings will get them out or throw up her hands in dismay and retreat.

Development is left on a cafeteria basis, with each person determining her own development needs. Performance review and evaluation are easy for a

1,1-oriented nursing administrator. With low standards for what is expected of others, performance review is tackled reluctantly and conducted in a very superficial manner.

Productivity is likely to sink to the lowest tolerable level. If it becomes mandatory to increase it, the solution is to employ more people—she is always short of staff—or purchase more equipment, thus increasing expense without resolving the basic problem.

Inertia is the rule when it comes to the introduction of change. The 1,1-oriented nursing administrator acts to initiate change only when under specific instructions to do so.

Chapter 6

THE 5,5-ORIENTED NURSING ADMINISTRATOR

The 5,5 orientation of the nurse administrator is in the middle of the Grid, where a moderate degree of concern for production is combined with a moderate degree of concern for those being supervised. This is the most frequently practiced theory of supervision in many institutions, and its popularity is growing, with many nurses knowing nothing better to do than to shift into a safe 5,5 orientation. We can get a sense of what the 5,5 orientation is all about by examining some well-known phrases: "A half loaf is better than none." "To get along, you've got to go along." "You scratch my back and I'll scratch yours." The common assumption underlying each of these is that while you do not go all the way to 9 on either of the Grid dimensions, neither do you take up the "couldn't-care-less" 1,1-oriented attitude. What you do is take the middle road of compromise, accommodation, and give-and-take, since you see it as the way everyone else does—neither more nor less.

The positive motivation of a 5,5-oriented nursing administrator is to belong:

"I want to look good, to be *in* with my colleagues."

She does this by seeking her sense of direction through finding out what the majority thinks or does. Being popular means putting together a package of qualities that are sought after in society, which includes whatever is fashionable in dress, neighborhoods to live in, places to go, books to read, and other forms of social expression. She is likely to develop pleasant manners and strive to become an interesting conversationalist. Her goal is to make many friends, even though not necessarily close ones.

A nursing administrator motivated by membership tends to be superficial in her own convictions. She avoids exposure by taking her cues from the actions of others. The prevailing opinions of others are her opinions; what others reject, she rejects. Therefore she is unlikely to have deep ideological commitments, whether political, religious, literary, social, institutional, or otherwise. She experiences a sense of well-being when evaluated positively by

65

fellow administrators and others. These good feelings may persist even though she may have just compromised a long-term gain for a short-term convenience. She may embrace a point of view only because her superiors and colleagues did so. She may have withheld a vital piece of information to avoid anticipated ostracism, or winked at a shady practice because "everybody else does it." The ability to back and fill, to shift and twist and turn, and yet stay with the majority is important to a 5,5-oriented nursing administrator's style. When she achieves the objective, the 5,5-oriented nurse feels okay. The motivational motto is:

"If I think, look, and act like everyone else, but a little more so, I will be a nursing administrator in good standing in the line to move up."

Viewed from the negative side of her motivation, she wants to avoid being a minority of one, separated from the mainstream, or becoming the object of ridicule, even though the position she stands for may in fact be a valid one.

Sometimes the 5,5-oriented nurse is unsuccessful and feels unpopular, out of step, and isolated from the "in" group. Being out of step can lead to censure and even loss of membership. Then she experiences a sense of shame whenever it becomes evident that she has lost social standing.

NURSE IN THE MIDDLE

The 5,5-oriented nursing administrator finds it easy to accommodate and adjust in her role between those above her and the staff members she supervises. She may see her role as that of a catalyst or facilitator in any situation she confronts. When uncertain about making a decision, she may "tease" guidance out of her superior without the superior recognizing her uncertainty. Then the 5,5-oriented nursing administrator can be seen as initiating and exercising responsibility, yet she does not get herself in a bind by deviating from what her superior says.

In the following example, Joyce Landon, the director of nurses, is tentatively feeling out the possibility of new shift changes with the hospital administrator.

In the coffee shop this morning, Joyce casually mentions to Ted Wells, the hospital administrator, that one of the staff nurses has proposed a new shift plan by which the nurses would work longer hours, but allow them more time off to be with their families. "It might not be a bad idea," Joyce continues, "Who couldn't use time off!"

"The problem around here, though, Joyce," replies Ted, "is that with the new wing going up, I don't want any more hassle right now. One more change is one too many."

"You're probably right, Ted. And besides, I don't think there is a hospital in the country doing what is being proposed." Joyce finishes her coffee and chats a little longer, knowing that Ted has ultimately made the decision for her.

Later she goes back and tells the staff nurse of her conversation with Mr. Wells, making sure that the staff nurse knows that Joyce will bring it up when the new wing is completed.

Joyce's handling of this situation is in the 5,5 orientation because she weighed the reactions to her feeler in terms of what Ted thought rather than the true merit of the proposal made by the staff nurse. Also, she had no precedent that she could think of on which to base any further consideration of the proposal.

ADMINISTRATIVE ASPECTS OF NURSING
Planning and scheduling

A 5,5 orientation to managing is responsive leadership. Many ways of moving forward, always in step with others and never in the lead, typify the approach. It stays within the bounds of what everyone else is doing as the ultimate criterion for appropriateness or pertinence. This amounts to a philosophy of gradualism where change is by trial and error or improvisation, not by goal-oriented direction or experiment. The result is neither chaotic nor coherent; it is more likely to be conformity centered and to come out piecemeal and makeshift.

According to this type of supervising, a nursing administrator does not command or direct to get the job done so much as she "motivates" and communicates. She avoids exerting formal authority. Her approach is to make requests in order to get her staff to want to work. Here is how the 5,5-oriented nursing administrator thinks of herself as a planner:

"I make plans according to what I know the staff members will accept and what they will reject. Then I plan for each staff nurse according to what she will think is okay."

Take the example of the responsibility of a head nurse to make out the daily assignments for her staff. She not only makes out the assignments but takes time to explain them. She also asks for the staff members' okay to make sure that they agree with her request. "I encourage them to feel free to come back if they don't like or understand what to do."

Maureen, head nurse in the following example, tries to approach an assignment indirectly. She tries to get her staff nurses to accept the solution to the problem in a mechanical manner so that no one is inconvenienced.

Maureen, head nurse, has just finished listening to the recording left by the night charge nurse, which has details on the burn patient admitted last night. Maureen finishes making notes and prepares to give the assignments to the staff.

"Listen," Maureen begins, "Mr. Lockman in 205 has third-degree burns over his abdomen and arms. He is also a diabetic and will have to be watched very closely by someone. We are short one nurse and Sylvia (the ward clerk) is ill today."

Several of the staff nurses offer suggestions, some complain about it not being possible to cover all patients adequately under this type of shortage.

"Well, I guess what we could do," decides Maureen, "is to take turns. Anne can take the first one since her name begins with A, Barbara the next one because her name begins with B. I'll be back up and relieve for coffee breaks. Maybe that will work."

This is a 5,5-oriented approach to planning and scheduling. Maureen is "testing the wind" and seeks a mechanical balance of the inconvenience so as not to upset someone.

Execution

Another responsibility is to see that the work assigned is being carried out. The 5,5-oriented nursing administrator checks up on each staff member. She does this by reviewing the progress each makes. If the staff nurse runs behind or has difficulty, the nursing administrator rearranges conditions wherever possible, adding a little help here, reducing assignments there, so that everything comes out acceptable and okay.

"I keep track of what the staff members are doing. If someone has difficulty, I try to reduce pressure by rearranging work assignments wherever possible."

Elizabeth, a head nurse, checks with Dan, an LPN, on his assignment. We see from this example a typical half-way approach in her manner of dealing with him.

Dan is leaning up against the wall of the hospital corridor with a look of puzzlement on his face. The assignment Elizabeth gave him was to bathe all the patients on the west side of the hall before doctors' rounds.

Elizabeth comes down the hall, sees Dan, and says, "What's the matter, Dan? You look awfully serious about something."

"Well, actually," said Dan, "I'm trying to figure out how I'm going to complete my assignment and get to my class on catheterizations on time."

"You are in a dilemma," laughs Elizabeth. "I guess you could get started with the baths and see how far you get. Or, I guess I could do some of them. Anyway, one person can't do everything at once, can they? At least you will have done some of the baths. That's better than nothing."

Elizabeth avoided being pushy or direct to get the job done, preferring to soften Dan's dilemma by urging him to settle what could be done with little inconvenience to him and no danger of any negative feedback to her.

Follow-up

The 5,5-oriented head nurse's approach to follow-up is to rely heavily on the checklist and the completion of the forms that signify that the procedures and techniques were carried out. The emphasis is more on the completion of the tasks that need to be done, and an indication by the nurse that the activity has been carried out, than ensuring that the activity itself was done in a thorough and thoughtful way. The paper system is what is concentrated upon, and the presumption might be made by the administrative nurse that when the paper is in order everything is okay. Thus, the importance attached to completing the checklist, for example, is to ensure that all of the staff nurses have completed those entries for which they are responsible. Equal with concern for the satisfactorily completed checklist, however, is concern for not putting the staff nurses under pressure if they are responsible for entries that are incomplete. Thus, the head nurse will ask them to complete it from memory rather than push the nurse to return to the patient and complete the procedure or technique.

In the following example, Rachel, head nurse, is willing to overlook Nell's forgetfulness on taking temperature.

All the nurses are at the station after the morning rounds doing charting. Nell, staff nurse, looks exasperated as she suddenly realizes that she forgot to take one of the patient's temperature.

"Why not see what yesterday's temperature was?" suggests Rachel. "Maybe you could put down something close to that or just put down normal if she's had no real variation the last three days. There's no sense in going to the trouble of taking it now. What matters is that you've got all the spaces checked."

This is a 5,5 approach to follow-up because Rachel is willing to overlook Nell's forgetfulness on the basis that it is too much trouble and the fact that completing the paperwork was the important thing at that point.

The flow of work through people is quite fragile; the 5,5 approach requires constant attention because it is a delicate balancing act, combined with the skills of a go-between. Her attitude might go something like this:

"I meet with the staff member involved in the assignment. I point out what she is doing right as well as what she is doing wrong without appearing critical. I also suggest, rather than actually *tell* her, how she can improve."

As you can see, Shelley's handling of the following situation is based on what she thinks about the circumstances rather than directly seeing that Mr. Richards is taken care of. Shelley is head nurse on the unit.

It is well into the morning and most of the staff nurses are doing charting. Some of the doctors have made their morning rounds. While waiting for others to come in, Shelley is visiting with one of the patients.

"Mrs. Bradshaw," inquired Mr. Richards, who is recovering from a leg amputation, "I understood the doctor to say that my dressing would be changed this morning."

"Yes, that's right. You mean it hasn't?" inquired Shelley.

Indeed, it hadn't and later Shelley approached the subject with Sue, the staff nurse responsible for Mr. Richard's care.

"I really haven't had time to do it," says Sue. "I spent a lot of time with Mrs. Grey who had the disc operation. She's such a lovely person to talk with and such fun, I just couldn't seem to get away. Is Mr. Richards uncomfortable?"

"Oh, no," responded Shelley. "He just felt that you would have been in by this time. Maybe you ought to go check on him when you have a minute."

Shelley comes through here as tentative in suggesting that Sue see Mr. Richards. No doubt Mr. Richards will continue to complain until finally some definite action is taken, perhaps by complaining to the doctor, or perhaps Sue will finally get her act together.

COMMUNICATION

Communication is extremely important to elicit suggestions from staff members and to consider their points of view. Under the 5,5 orientation to nursing administration, just about equal weight is given to formal communication as to the informal network.

A 5,5-oriented nursing administrator does not command or direct, but suggests. She motivates and communicates to get the job done. The 5,5-oriented leadership style is to request and to sell—to try to get people to want to work by staying a half step ahead. The nursing administrator tests an order by explaining why it is needed and by seeing if people will buy it. She reasons, "People will go along if you tell them the reason something has to be done and let them talk and even gripe a little. That way they let off steam."

The informal level of communication involves the grapevine—rumors and heresay, as well as a good deal of irrelevant talk that is not pertinent to organization purpose. This includes everything from discotheque, social and sports events, to local political developments.

The nursing administrator's interest in informal communication is that it is an open window, the pulse of the staff members, how they are feeling, what is disturbing them, pressure points that worry them, and so on. By knowing the score on all these things, the 5,5-oriented nurse is in a position to take or recommend many different kinds of action. She can start a contradictory rumor in order to block one that needs to be countered. She can use what is known from the informal communication network as the basis for timing either good or bad "formal" messages from above. Beyond that, of course, by keeping in touch, she frequently is able to pass information upstairs that permits higher levels of hospital administration to take corrective action concerning matters that would have a bad effect if left unattended. Nothing about this informal communication is official, and it is likely to be indefinite as to who said what to whom: "They are saying. . ." "Everyone seems to know. . ." "Several of my people have mentioned in passing that. . . ."

In terms of what is being said among people, and what other people are eager to know, the 5,5-oriented nursing administrator is in the go-between position. She keeps herself tuned in to what is going on and tries to figure out what the public relations consequences will be if the decision is made to go that way. By a series of adjustments and corrections, the 5,5-oriented nursing administrator can find a position that gets the job done in a reasonably good manner without stirring up too much trouble.

Ruth, the head nurse in the following example, both sends and receives her communication through the informal grapevine.

One of the staff nurses, Suzy, approaches Ruth and says, "Ruth, have you done anything about replacing Ann-Marie and Jo Ann when they leave? I heard the other day that someone applied for a position but the personnel director told them the hospital wasn't hiring until September—two months away."

Ruth sighed. "Well, I haven't heard that, although I was told by one of the other head nurses to be prepared for some overtime until administration could get budgeting done. Who told you about not replacing personnel?"

"Barbara did," replied Suzy. "We've been wondering what's going to be done. It's only three more weeks until they leave."

"Oh," says Ruth, "I was getting around to it. In fact, I had mentioned it to the director of nurses and just haven't submitted the request. I guess I had better check and see what the situation actually is. I'll get the word around then. I will need to see how people feel about overtime."

Here we see that Ruth takes no specific action to include her staff members in discussing personnel plans for the unit. Rather, any information they get has been carried down by word of mouth. Ruth receives her information in the same manner, resulting in her communicating a great majority of the time in a tentative, unsure manner.

As might be expected from what has been said about communication, the 5,5-oriented head nurse avoids pinpointing specific directions to get the work done. To escape from being seen as pushy or demanding, she requests and tries to persuade and sell. It is a soft sell, without being too soft. Further, she throws out suggestions in a tentative manner to see what kinds of reactions people have. If they buy it, well and good; if they object, the manner of being tentative about what has been said makes it possible to back off and test another course of action without her losing face. Her attitude is:

"You have to keep your antenna out to know what is going on, that is, to get the signal."

Lee, head nurse, feels compelled to "test" the feelings of the majority to determine the acceptability of a new plan rather than evaluate its merits and convince others of the soundness of the new method.

The director of nurses, Helen Thompson, mentions to Lee that consideration is being given to developing a new department for discharge planning. Nothing is definite, however; it is still in the discussion stage.

"How do you suppose this will affect my staff?" Lee asks Helen. "I guess I really ought to check out their feelings about this rather than spring it on them when it's adopted. After all, I don't think anything like this has ever been tried here at Memorial, has it?"

"No, I don't think so," replies Helen.

In the early afternoon, two nurses approach Lee concerning the new department they have heard about. One complains, "Why do we need another department? Aren't we doing okay the way we are?

Lee explains, "Well, Administration seems to think it would be better if one person were responsible for discharge planning."

Another staff nurse volunteers, "Personally, I like the idea. That's one less thing I have to worry about."

Now Lee doesn't really know how to react except to say that maybe she should check with each of the other nurses and see how they feel. Then she can get back with the director of nurses.

Lee's handling of this situation is in the 5,5 orientation because she thinks in terms of meeting informally with each nurse rather than bringing people together to think through the concept.

CONFLICT

The 5,5 approach is based upon a easygoing kind of logic. It says, "What person or movement has ever had its exclusive way? Extreme positions promote conflict and they certainly should be avoided. Experience shows, again and again, that steady progress comes from compromise and a willingness to yield some advantages in order to gain others."

A 5,5-oriented conflict resolution runs the gamut, with the nursing administrator utilizing whatever technique she thinks will be needed to bring conflict to an acceptable end.

In everyday usage, diplomacy and tact refer to 5,5-oriented kinds of actions because they are calculated to avoid conflict by structuring the relationships to

people and their interactions according to preset rules. Though many are un-
stated, they are widely understood.

From a 5,5 perspective, it is seldom wise to confront conflict directly, even
when the circumstances are self-evident. The reason is that someone wins and
someone loses. Many conflicts represent the hot emotion of the moment. It is
best to back off, to let the situation cool. Breathing time provides the chance to
find the middle ground. Sometimes the 5,5-oriented nursing administrator is
caught in a situation of conflict where the position she has been responsible for
is wrong, but to admit it, she thinks, would cause her to lose status. Bending
the truth, half truths, or white lies all may be useful to effect the face-saving
resolution. Over a period of time, however, such distortions are likely to form a
patchwork of contradictions, reversals, starts and stops, and so forth. Yet the
5,5-oriented nursing administrator feels that this is the practical or realistic
approach to management: one that can get a job done without stirring up too
much trouble. When conflict arises, the question often is not what is best, but
what is the politically safe, salable, or workable solution.

When two subordinates are in conflict, a 5,5-oriented nursing administrator may separate them and talk with each one individually. Then she tries to
find points on which they both can agree. She suggests her proposal to each
one separately. This is likely to result in some basis of agreement that each
subordinate can live with, even though they may continue to dislike one another. If the conflict persists, planning for them to work different days or shifts
may reduce the conflict or, as a last resort, she may arrange for one of them to be
transferred. This is depicted in the following situation.

Joan, a staff nurse, stops and says to the head nurse, Beth, "Please do something
about Frieda and Beverly. They are always fighting and it is difficult working with
them."

Later on, Beth meets Beverly and says to her, "What's this about Frieda. I understand she bothers you. What's wrong?"

Beverly says, "I can't take Frieda any more. She's lazy and never helps out. She does
her own work and leaves as soon as she gives her patients' reports to the night people. I
can't get her to listen, so I explode at her."

Beth decides to hear Frieda's side, and Frieda says, "That Beverly, she just gets
worked up over nothing. I do my work and I do leave because I have to get home so the
babysitter can go home. If I keep her longer, I have to pay double time. There isn't
that much to do, but I'm sure it's because I leave that it's like a bull with a red flag. Don't
put us together. I have a headache every time I get home."

Beth knows the best way to handle this would be to transfer one to another unit, but
there is no guarantee that she would get a replacement. Besides, they are both good
workers and she likes them. She decides on a compromise and tells them, "When
evening time is made out, I'll try and not put you on together. However, for the times
when I have to, do you think you could try and work things out?"

Beth handles the conflict between Frieda and Beverly in a 5,5-oriented manner. She talks to each one separately and concludes that they do in fact have a conflict. Thereafter, she tries to find an administrative way around the situation by separating them for their assignment times whenever possible. The goal is to reduce the tension between them by having them not work at the same time. She meets with each one separately and pleads with each to try to get along during those unavoidable times when they both work on the same day. Her additional implicit assumption is that, if they are not together for a period of time, the hostile feelings between them will cool off, and thereafter they should be able to work okay together.

Mistakes and errors

The 5,5-oriented nursing administrator knows that no subordinate ever intended to make a mistake and appreciates that people are embarrassed when they have to admit having made one. Therefore, she gives the staff member the benefit of the doubt, at least initially. Her attitude might be stated this way:

"So you made a mistake. So what! Everyone makes one now and then. Perhaps you could double check that type of procedure before you try it again. What do you think?"

The 5,5-oriented nursing administrator approach, then, for managing mistakes and errors is first of all to keep the tempo at an acceptable pace so that people are not under pressure. If a mistake occurs, she will try to give the staff member the benefit of the doubt or overlook it if possible. Finally, the nursing administrator encourages subordinates to work according to rules, traditions, precedents, and long-established past practices. This is not necessarily literally, but in the sense of staying close enough so that shortcuts that might produce mistakes and errors can be avoided. Then, if something does go wrong, the nursing administrator at least has the possibility of avoiding criticism from her superiors.

Furthermore, a 5,5-oriented nursing administrator is as embarrassed as anyone if it becomes necessary to admit that mistakes are being made because of failure to follow rules and procedures. As a result, the nursing administrator is likely to stick to the rules and will want her staff to do the same. Then, if a mistake does occur, at least she will not be blamed for exercising too little control over performance deviation. However, this shows that the 5,5-oriented nursing administrator is almost more concerned about keeping herself blameless than about reducing errors and mistakes.

Because of this devotion to the "book," organizations managed in a 5,5-oriented way are quite bureaucratic. People have learned the importance of closely adhering to rules, regulations, and red tape to avoid blame, rather than to use these guidelines as they were intended: to give guidance and, if rigid or irrelevant, to gain permission to disregard them or to work openly to get them repealed or changed.

Rebecca, head nurse, handles errors in ordering supplies in a 5,5-oriented way. She knows that the problem lies with Marian, the unit manager, but rather than try to get to the root of the problem and find a valid solution, she "requests" her better effort in hopes that managing the symptoms will take care of the mistakes.

On two occasions during the last month, a supply order had been filled out wrong, resulting in costly interim orders having to be made. Today it happened again.

Rebecca, head nurse, approaches the new unit manager, Marian, who is responsible for ordering supplies.

Clearing her throat to get Marian's attention she begins, "Marian, we need to watch the supply orders a little closer. Mr. Northrup complained to me last week about expenses. We all need to be a little more careful. I know you are doing a good job and are really trying hard. No doubt you have things on your mind. But I would appreciate your paying a little more attention."

"Oh, another thing done wrong! Will I ever learn this job!"

Exasperated, Marian jumps up from her desk and leaves Rebecca standing there. Rebecca watches Marian as she runs down the hall, head bent, hands shielding her eyes.

"I feel sorry for her," Rebecca says to herself, "but I had to check her before things got worse."

Rebecca visits several patients, which keeps her from returning to the nurses' station for some time. She doesn't want to risk seeing Marian any more that afternoon.

This is a 5,5-oriented approach to managing mistakes because Rebecca gives only surface treatment to what evidently is a work problem aggravated by a more deep-seated human problem. She does not make an effort to find out what it is and simply assumes that Marian's thoughtlessness is the cause of the problem. Instead, she speaks to her about it in a tentative way that Marian accepts as a reprimand.

Complaints

The 5,5-oriented nursing administrator is supersensitive to complaints. They are disturbing because they signal troubles the staff members are having that can impede production and reduce her popularity. They can also result in the nursing administrator being criticized by her supervisor for being ineffective in solving the staff's problems as they affect morale. Realizing that failure to deal with them can have a bad effect on steady, continuing productivity that is wanted, a 5,5-oriented nursing administrator responds to complaints. She believes in the "open door" policy, even though she is not crazy about the idea. Everyone has direct access for discussions in private on a topic at any time. In this way the 5,5-oriented nursing administrator shows concern. When they come for discussion, however, it tends to be brief and superficial; real problems are not tackled.

Some complaints are difficult to deal with because they refer to matters over which the nursing administrator has no control, or which, if taken higher up, would place her popularity at risk. When a complaint is lodged, she is likely to talk it over with the staff and help perceive the complaint in a different light. When looked at from another angle, the problem does not appear as important as it had appeared previously. Leaving things as is and getting people to accept them is the 5,5-oriented administrator's basic approach to dealing with complaints.

When this approach does not work, her tendency is to move in a tentative way and say, "Let me take it up with my superior and see if anything can be done about it." Then if she comes back with partial success, perhaps a concession can be provided to the staff member, who in turn can feel that some progress is made. "Half a loaf is better than none" is frequently quoted by the 5,5-oriented nursing administrator, and she can take credit for making the effort to solve the problem.

Another strategy for dealing with complaints is to bargain. The head nurse might say, "Look, I am really sorry that you have to work overtime. That is something I can't do anything about. However, there is something I can do that I believe will be helpful, and I would like to do it as a personal favor to make up for the difficulty you are in."

By being available to people and responding to a complaint if possible, or blunting its sharpness by compromising and bargaining, a 5,5-oriented nursing administrator is often—but not always—able to create a "live and let live" kind of climate.

In the following example, we see how the head nurse, Mary, responds to a patient's complaint about Judy, the staff nurse, in a 5,5-oriented way.

One of the patients, Rosy Crowther, has requested to see the head nurse, Mary. Rosy says, "I'm sorry to complain, but please don't assign Judy Hester to take care of me any more. She's very nervous and jittery, and talks and talks and talks. She talks so much she gives me a headache."

Mary says, "Let me see what I can do. I'll take care of it for you."

She goes out of the room, and as she goes down the corridor she thinks, "This is not the first complaint I've had about Judy, and if I don't do something to solve the problem at once, it's going to rub off on me and my reputation."

She recalls that this morning another head nurse, Roberta, on 7 West, mentioned that she was short of staff. She wonders if she might recommend to the director of nurses that Judy be transferred to Roberta.

The transfer is arranged in a magnanimous "gesture" to help another unit in its time of distress. Now Roberta has the needed help, and it is her patients, not Mary's, who are likely to be doing the complaining.

Mary will be asking for additional help to ease her "burden" in due course, and the merry-go-round will have completed another turn.

We can anticipate that Roberta will have to eventually face the same dilemma with Judy and her talkativeness, but as for Mary, she has failed to "foot the problem."

Hostile feelings

Hostile feelings are worrisome to a 5,5-oriented nursing administrator. They cause her anxiety and she does not think well under the emotional pressure that is involved. One reason is that, to balance production and people concerns, the nursing administrator feels the need for stable conditions. When hostility erupts, it is as though the ground beneath her equilibrium scales is trembling and threatening to throw her off balance.

How does a 5,5-oriented nursing administrator react when a staff member expresses hostile feelings? She may do any one or more of several things, but they all are based on similar, if not identical, assumptions regarding how to moderate, reduce, or eliminate bad feelings.

The first attempt may be to keep the conversation fairly superficial so that the staff member does not have the opportunity to become upset. For example, the nursing administrator attempts to focus the conversation on operational matters and away from personalities. Second, she does her best to avoid expressing hostile feelings toward the staff member because, if she did, the discussion might become a win-lose fight, and that kind of battle is definitely something she wants to avoid. Third, if a staff member is very angry, the nursing administrator might try to appease her and make a move to create a cooling off period, during which time she can think over what to do. She says, "I very much appreciate your telling me these things. They are important to me, but rather than give you a quick reaction, I would like to think these things over. Could we get together next Monday?" By using this strategy, the nursing administrator not only gains time to think, but also chances are the staff member will calm down during the interim. Thus, when they get back together the emotion of the moment will have died away, or if it has not, at least the nursing administrator is in a position to offer the staff member alternative ways of thinking about the problem. This is really a splitting technique. It has in it much of the same basic thinking as in other 5,5-oriented nursing administrator techniques that involve compromise, adjustment, and accommodation of differences.

Barbara is the head nurse in the following example. Her 5,5 approach is to acknowledge the hostile feelings, but her goal is to relieve the tensions rather than to get to the core of the problem, which evidently she can do something about.

Marge, Grace, and Dot, all staff nurses, are angry. They feel like they have been put down since the LPN, Bernice, gets all the interesting patients and better time, or so it seems to them. Evidently they think Bernice is the head nurse's favorite person. Bernice has been there longer than all the RN's.

The staff nurses confront Barbara. "Something has to be done. We can't work like this any longer. We've had it. You treat Bernice much better than you do us, and we don't like it. So don't expect us to take it any longer."

Barbara, a little taken aback, says, "Oh, now, wait a minute. Let's talk about this a little. You really *are* upset. Surely one person can't get all three of you so angry."

"It's her attitude, Barbara," says Marge. "She thinks she has it made around here."

"Okay," Barbara replies. "Why don't you cool down a little and we'll meet back on this, say tomorrow about one o'clock." The nurses agree and leave, their anger cooled for the time being.

As they walk away, Grace, speaking to Marge and Dot, says, "Thank goodness we got it off our chests and out in the open," adding, "I feel better already, don't you?"

In the meantime Barbara gives Bernice a few of the more undesirable patients and assignments. Now at the one o'clock meeting she can demonstrate impartiality.

This is a temporary solution, of course, not a permanent one, and we can expect that Bernice will soon enjoy favored treatment again.

DEVELOPMENT

When a 5,5-oriented nursing administrator has a say in the selection of staff, she makes sure that they fit in with the other staff members; that is, that they are all compatible. She prefers an extended orientation program. During the orientation time, rules, regulations, policies, procedures, mechanics of pay and vacation, and so forth are presented and discussed in detail. Usually the effort given to development is only lip service, more focused on getting people to accept the expected routines than on developing their nursing skills and capabilities. As a result, formalized programs are designed to reinforce hospital positions, policies, and procedures to make the new staff person more knowledgeable of the organization and how to use it to get the work done rather than to aid her to learn new professional skills. Her attitude is: "I seek people who will fit in."

In the following example, Nelda, head nurse, is explaining the orientation program to Polly, a new graduate, recently employed on 2 South.

"For the first month, Polly," Nelda is saying, "I'll put you with a 'buddy' so that you can learn the system, the doctors, and so forth. I might warn you about Dr. Williams. He's very peculiar, so the best thing to do is not to question him; just do as he wishes. You will also learn that we have a number of forms to complete on this unit. It is something you learn to put up with. It's been done that way for as long as I have been here."

"How many nurses are on this unit?" ventures Polly.

"Sixteen, and they all get along very well. If you have any problems with anyone, just try to stay on their good sides. That way no real problems will crop up."

Nelda's primary concern was that Polly would be an unsettling influence on the unit. In her 5,5-oriented way, Nelda cautions her to accept things as they are and go along to get along with the other nurses.

The 5,5-oriented approach to performance review and evaluation can well be called the "sandwich" technique. A "good" comment is introduced before a negative one in order to promote good feelings. This is followed by a discussion of a few improvement steps so that the whole process is characterized as being more or less acceptable to the staff member. In other words, the nursing administrator prepares in advance for a performance review and, then, having clearly in mind what to say, begins by saying something positive about the staff member's performance. Then she brings up a negative point stated in the best possible way, followed by a complimentary evaluation. In this way, whatever "sting" the negative evaluation might contain will be taken out by the two positives.

"I tend to emphasize good points and avoid appearing critical, though I do encourage staff members to identify their own weak points."

Although Jocelyn, the head nurse, knows that Mae's performance as LPN is unsatisfactory, she carefully avoids doing something about it. She does, however, "request" some improvement in the period ahead.

Mae, LPN, has made errors in the past which resulted in incident reports being written up in her file. It is now the day of her semiannual evaluation and she is sitting beside the head nurse, Jocelyn, discussing her performance.

"As far as that medication error is concerned, Jocelyn," Mae explains, "it really wasn't my fault. Evidently when Dr. Ball dictated the order to me, I wrote it down wrong."

"You may have a point there, and we've no way to check it out anyway," replies Jocelyn. "I suppose you shouldn't feel too badly about it." Jocelyn pauses and then continues, "You and Dr. Ball get along quite well, otherwise, don't you?"

"Oh, yes, quite well," says Mae, "and about those other incidents, well, you know what a strain I've been under with the divorce and all."

Jocelyn appears thoughtful and then responds, "I understand, and I think overall you are doing okay. Perhaps you ought to be more careful and not have to write any more incident reports for a while, don't you think? With the divorce over there will be less tension for sure. Then we'll talk more about it later on and see if everything's okay. Is that all right with you?"

This is a 5,5 orientation of the sort that takes a weak explanation of the problem at face value on a "let's see if it works" basis. Jocelyn is indirect in getting to the real source of Mae's problem. It is a wishy-washy method of putting up with a less-than-satisfactory performance in anticipation of its becoming better tomorrow.

INTRODUCTION OF CHANGE

The attitude toward change under a 5,5 orientation is that it is inevitable but should not be disruptive. Therefore, change should be introduced in a series of steps rather than in one fell swoop. The reason for this lower, more evolutionary approach is that the status quo retains its basic features, and the change comes as a series of patches on the status quo rather than any dramatic or basic change taking place in the status quo operation itself. In this way, no one is disrupted, and staff members can continue doing the same things they were previously doing but with slight alterations or modifications. It is unnecessary, in other words, for people to learn an entirely new way of operating.

In the following example, the 5,5-oriented director of nurses is discussing with a head nurse how to introduce the unit manager with a minimum of resistance.

The head nurse says, "Oh, no! Do I have to have another person in my area? Things are bad enough as it is. What will he do?"

The director of nurses says, "The unit manager will take care of all those housekeeping type duties—things that you've been yelling about for years, such as broken equipment, housekeeping functions, dietary, and so on. You can keep the nursing activities such as ordering drugs and taking off orders from doctors' order books. We'll put him someplace where he won't be in your way. How's that? Will you do it? I'm trying to see if it will work. If it is successful on your unit, I'll try it on others. If it isn't, I will have to shelve the whole idea."

The head nurse reluctantly says, "Well, we'll try it and see how it works out."

In the preceding example, the director of nurses has a 5,5 orientation because she allows a gradual introduction of the use of the unit manager. She avoids confronting the head nurse with her attitude about having to give up the "status" activities of the head nurse. In this sense, the status quo is essentially retained, with a small degree of shift of some of the duties to an additional person on the unit. It is the director of nurse's attitude that, if things go well, it will be possible to remove some of the other activities gradually.

REACTIONS TO 5,5 SUPERVISION

Staff members rarely react negatively to being managed in a 5,5-oriented way because, on the surface, it is so reasonable. Yet this approach to leadership leaves much to be desired.

Like begets like

The prospect is that, under a 5,5 orientation, a staff nurse comes to think or manage in the same way she is being managed. Because actions are reasonable in the sense of "live and let live," it is to be expected that the nursing administrator and her staff will move along in a steady-paced way, not really involved in the pursuit of excellence, and yet doing a more or less acceptable job. Over the long term, sharp edges are rubbed off, individual ambitions are modified, patients come to be taken somewhat for granted, and things move along.

Playing the game

Once immersed in a 5,5-oriented system, a staff member may enjoy the status game and refine her skills for staying within it, describing her life and work in this fashion:

"I like things as they are and figure the hospital will reward me by promotion because of my loyalty and steady service and popularity with everyone."

This acceptance of the status quo with its conventional values, status symbols, and steady progress through seniority, popularity, and reasonableness is a 5,5 response to a 5,5 environment. It is an uncomplicated approach characterized by accommodation and adjustment. Commitment demands no effort beyond staying up with or maybe just a little ahead of the pack. To challenge the status quo is a jarring element and is to be avoided. Therefore, no one in a 5,5 organization is prepared to challenge the system. If they want to stay, they must abide by the organization's rules. One such rule is to always ask, "What will those above me accept?" Then the nursing administrator puts forward a request that she knows the agency will find acceptable.

Drifting into 1,1

Another reaction is from those who want to contribute more but find their efforts unrewarded, unappreciated, and even sidetracked by the 5,5-oriented nursing administrator's way of running the unit. If unprepared to leave the hospital for another position, or unable to afford to leave, they are likely to drift slowly into 1,1 as a reaction from doing the same things again and again until they are dull and boring. Nursing then becomes a ritual or a retreat from involvement.

SUMMARY

A 5,5 orientation as a supervisory approach is when the nursing administrator adjusts to the system and accepts whatever tempo others have come to adopt, as long as it is reasonable. She does not push for more even though results obtained are less than what might have been accomplished by a different approach to supervision. Tradition, precedent, and past practice, policies, and procedures are relied on. When differences do arise between the nursing administrator and her staff members, they are relieved to the extent possible by splitting the difference in ways that include compromise, accommodation, and adjustment. In terms of specific elements of management, the 5,5 orientation can be summarized as follows.

A 5,5-oriented nursing administrator is interested in and attentive to problems of management that can be solved by thoughtful communication. She realizes that a supervisor between higher levels and lower levels is a go-between, responsible for passing information up about subordinate morale, attitudes, feelings, and concerns, as well as passing management concerns down. The 5,5-oriented nursing administrator uses the formal communication channels in terms of such things as regular meetings and memoranda, but also pays close attention to informal communication, examples of which are rumors, the grapevine, and complaints. The goal, through effective communication, is to anticipate difficulties and in this way to avoid them.

Planning and scheduling is of a general character. In this way, staff members are unlikely to feel excessive pressure. The nursing administrator is available to give help whenever staff members feel the need and request it. In this easy give-and-take way, performance is accomplished, not necessarily at a high level, but to an acceptable degree.

Conflict is avoided. Mistakes and errors are seen as inevitable, but if they are not handled in a "sound" manner, acrimony and antagonism can result. One way of avoiding mistakes is to encourage staff members to work according to long-established practices or as set down in operating manuals, not to the literal letter, but within appropriate guidelines. In this way, errors from shortcuts are avoided, although gains from discovering innovative practices are sacrificed. At first, and for a limited number of repeats of the same mistake, the 5,5-oriented nursing administrator gives staff members the benefit of the doubt.

Reacting to complaints is a very delicate matter, and the 5,5-oriented nursing administrator seeks ways of keeping emotions from erupting. She may attempt to do this by channeling a discussion into administrative areas or by introducing cooling-off periods that provide time to think and that also allow the hostile feelings to fade.

Change is introduced on a step-at-a-time basis so that the impact of any reactions can be carefully gauged. The nursing administrator adjusts or postpones any further activity if she feels that her membership is threatened. Otherwise, however, any effort to change things has patchwork characteristics because of her accommodation to what others want.

Orientation is done in such a manner that the new staff member is well indoctrinated as to the policies and procedures of the hospital agency. More emphasis is placed on formalized programs than on learning professional skills. Performance evaluation is carried out in such a manner as to get the staff member to acknowledge her faults and promise to rectify them. In this way the nursing administrator avoids being openly critical, because the staff member is unlikely to feel that the nursing administrator is holding her to the line about those matters that the staff member has admitted represent unsatisfactory performance up to now. Otherwise, sandwich techniques of embedding criticism between complaints are employed to take the sting away.

The 5,5 orientation to supervision is based on a safe and widely used set of assumptions and related techniques for keeping things moving at a steady pace. It is safe because it does get people to "perform," not to a high degree, but in an acceptable range, and it does avoid people problems—though again, not entirely. It is a fairly successful way of keeping production-people requirements on an even keel if, as belief has it, "too much" of one means "too little" of the other.

Chapter 7

THE 9,9-ORIENTED NURSING ADMINISTRATOR

The 9,9 Grid style is in the upper right corner of the Grid figure where a 9 of concern for results is joined with a 9 of concern for people. It is the theory that says, "Through active participation of staff members, their involvement and commitment to find and apply the best solutions in everyday work can be earned. Those who are supervised in a 9,9 way want to win, and the measure of winning is that results are truly excellent."

The nursing administrator's 9,9 achievement motivation comes from developing the competency required to make a positive contribution. She pursues goals and objectives that are simultaneously personal and organizational. There is a sense of gratification, enthusiasm, and excitement from making an important contribution. The closer one comes to success, the greater the sense of emotional reward.

When an effort fails, a 9,9-oriented nursing administrator is likely to feel self-defeat, disappointment, and discouragement. She may be disturbed or uneasy, faced with self-doubt about her ability to meet future problems successfully. Setbacks occur but perspective provides the foundation for persistence. Failure in the short term is not the end of everything. The motivational motto is, "What is worth doing is worth doing well."

The 9,9 orientation to supervision takes more skill, personal leadership, and teamwork than do the other Grid styles. The nursing administrator is a leader in four ways. First, she helps staff members to see possibilities that might not otherwise be recognized. Second, she is also a leader in fully utilizing the resources that subordinates are able to contribute in achieving such goals. Third, she uses development strategies so that those she supervises can expand their capacities. Fourth, this style of leadership aids people to set high goals of the kind that are attainable only through committed effort, and sometimes only through learning new skills essential for success.

In all other Grid styles—9,1, 1,9, 5,5, 1,1 and maternalism—concern for people and concern for production (results) are seen as mutually exclusive. As an example, a nursing administrator in a 9,1 orientation might say, "I've got to have better results, and I must put more pressure on my people." A 1,9-oriented administrator says, "We put less pressure on our people and, while production has not improved, everyone seems happier and more at ease." A 5,5-oriented nursing administrator looks through her bifocals and tries to accommodate and compromise to try to get balance on both sides, staying a half-step ahead of the status quo, hoping for improvements one small step after another. A 1,1-oriented administrator hides from problems because she does not want to see them. All of these take for granted an either/or or a neither attitude. They set up a false assumption and then abide by its indications. Drop the assumption that high concern for results inevitably cancels out high concern for people, and what do you get? The two high concerns can be unified into an entirely new way of leading. This is where 9,9 takes off.

Behavioral science laws of human participation must be respected to ensure sound supervision that integrates production and people concerns. Each of the following statements is consistent with a 9,9 orientation, and is supported in research evidence from social psychology, sociology, anthropology, mental health, counseling, psychiatry, political science, history, and field studies of business effectiveness, as well as validated in reverse in studies of criminology, penology, colonialism, slavery, indentured servitude, and so on. Other things being equal, productivity, creativity, mental and physical health, and personal satisfaction are better served when:

- Fulfillment through contribution is the motivation that gives character to human activity and supports productivity.
- Mutual trust and respect undergird productive human relationships.
- Open communication supports mutual understanding.
- Activities carried out within a framework of goals and objectives integrate personal with organization goals.
- Conflict resolution by direct problem-solving confrontation promotes personal health.
- Responsibility for one's own actions stimulates initiative.
- Efforts are applied to jobs that involve complex work activities or to a variety of simpler activities.
- Critique is used to learn from experience.

These generalizations appear to be true regardless of time, place, situation, race, religion or creed. Taken together, these statements represent different facets of a 9,9-oriented leadership style. Each reflects, in its own way, the basic proposition that there is one best way to supervise.

A point to be emphasized is about 9,9-oriented teamwork. Teamwork does *not* mean that all members must work physically together within sight and sound range of one another all the time. Far from it. For example, suppose a team has four members. Ann is the head nurse, and Stephanie, Cathy, and Cheryl are staff members. Some team problems involve only Ann—or only Stephanie and Cathy or Cheryl—in finding and in implementing the solution. Then it is in the interest of teamwork for the individual members to solve the problem alone, and the effectiveness of doing so contributes to teamwork by avoiding duplication of effort. Some team problems, in other words, are "one-alone."

Other problems involve only Ann and Stephanie together, but not Cathy or Cheryl. Since Cathy and others can contribute nothing to the solution, it is up to Ann and Stephanie to work out the solution between themselves. These one-to-one circumstances make it possible to free others who can contribute nothing to use their own time and effort dealing with their own solo responsibilities and assignments.

Some problems, however, can only be solved by Ann, Stephanie, Cathy, and Cheryl working out a situation as a unit. Such team situations are one-to-all.

Those who have tried the 9,9 way of supervision find it to be the best management style overall, whether the problem is solo, one-to-one, or one-to-all.

NURSE IN THE MIDDLE

It soon becomes evident, as one looks at the 9,9 orientation, that the two concerns can be unified so that the nursing administrator does not have to play one side against the other or try to stay in the middle, or escape. Both concerns come together in a unified way when people work together in solving problems through insight, creativity, and commitment.

In the following example, Madelyn Greenberg, director of nurses, approaches a change in work load. She approaches Norma, the maternity head, to help resolve the dilemma concerning temporary help.

Two years ago the board of trustees at West Central Hospital approved the addition of a new birthing center in the maternity ward. This center allows the mother-to-be to check in before the time of birth. A private room is designed much like an ordinary bedroom, with separate bath, facilities for the baby, and a kitchenette. The objective is to allow the mother to experience childbirth in as homelike and comfortable a manner as possible. The father is included in the care and feeding of the child after delivery.

The center is complete, with a grand opening scheduled for next week. Prominent women in the city have been invited to spend one night in the center as an extra measure of publicity in letting the public know about these facilities.

The problem this presents for Madelyn is that staff nurses will have to be temporarily transferred to the birthing center from other wards until the specialists hired can come on board.

Madelyn has called a meeting with the maternity head nurse, Norma. She explains that the birthing center will require two additional staff nurses and one LPN probably for about two weeks. She asks Norma if she has anyone she can spare.

"I don't know, Madelyn," Norma responds, "my floor is really tight right now. However, there is a possibility of Grace working overtime. She really needs the money. She could work an extra four hours if someone could be found to take the remaining time."

"Actually," Norma continues, "there is another alternative. This might be an excellent opportunity for the graduate nurses at the nursing college across the street to get some experience. Do you think the board would approve?"

"I think so," says Madelyn. "That's a good idea. I'll meet with Dr. Jansen tomorrow and doublecheck. If everything is okay, I'll draw up a schedule and present it to the director at the school. Would you talk with Grace and let me know if she would like this opportunity for overtime? Let me know as soon as you have the chance to check her out. Then we can get together and go over everything. If not, we'll have to study the situation again. We would like this new center to go without a hitch."

This is a 9,9 approach because Madelyn involved the maternity head nurse in arriving at a decision as to the next steps in getting the necessary help for the new birthing center. She is enthusiastic in listening to Norma's ideas. She also makes plans for meeting again to work out new alternatives if these tactics do not work.

ADMINISTRATIVE ASPECTS OF NURSING

We can now look at the basic areas of nursing administration.

Planning and scheduling

A 9,9-oriented nursing administrator thinks:

"Based on mutual understanding and agreement as to what the agency goals are and the means by which they are to be obtained, it is my job to make decisions, but it is equally important to see to it that sound decisions are made."

In a real sense, people and production are intertwined since decisions only strengthen patient care when those involved want the decision to be successful. The nursing administrator with a 9,9 orientation views her responsibility as seeing to it that planning and scheduling are accomplished in a sound way. There is no abdication of the 1,1 variety, no yielding of the kind that crops up under 1,9, no middle-of-the-road compromises as in 5,5, and no 9,1 masterminding. In the 9,9 approach, others who must implement plans are drawn in on the actual planning of work activities. The attitude might be expressed in this way:

"I get the reactions and ideas of staff members who have relevant facts or stakes in the outcome. Then, based on shared understanding, I establish schedules, procedures, and ground rules, and set up individual responsibilities."

This concept of participation is based on the notion that when staff members can influence outcomes, they support rather than comply or resist. Leadership that can arouse sound participation increases the probability that solutions achieved will be fundamentally sound, making constant review and revision unnecessary. People are able to give the best of themselves rather than seek the best for themselves as is often true when one's contributions are not sought.

What are the more specific characteristics of a 9,9 orientation in planning and scheduling? In the following example, Lydia, head nurse, takes a carefully thought out approach to finding the root cause of the patient's problem.

Lydia is head nurse on an obstetrical unit. Natalie, a staff nurse, has come to her about one of the new mothers, Rachel, who has been quite upset since the birth of her baby. Several times during the past two days she has become so angry with the staff over minor incidents that it is evident something is bothering her deeply.

In planning the assignments that day, Lydia and Natalie discuss Rachel and decide that Natalie will spend some time with her to find out just what the problem is.

Later Natalie finds out that Rachel is concerned about the baby because of a couple of bruises on its head. No one, including the doctor, has assured her the baby is okay. She is afraid to ask because she thinks something might be wrong. She thinks the baby's head might have been damaged in birth. She had often heard of cases where this had happened.

Natalie assures her nothing is wrong with the baby and promises to doublecheck with the doctor for her.

That afternoon Lydia and Natalie write up a report for the charge nurses of the other two shifts so that they are aware of the problem and what is being done.

"And also," Lydia and Natalie indicate in the report, "we'll be in touch in the next twenty-four hours to keep tab on progress and to see if we need to do anything differently before Rachel goes home."

This is a 9,9 approach because at the one-to-one level Lydia takes an active part in helping with the problem by okaying additional time for Natalie to dig in and find out what is behind the problem. Furthermore, both Natalie and Lydia recognize the importance of clueing in the charge nurses of the other two shifts on what is going on. They also set up a time to doublecheck in order to become as informed as possible as to Rachel's developing situation.

This illustration also helps us see that the charge nurses are as much a part of the nursing team as are Lydia and Natalie, even though they may not be able to get together physically.

Execution

Seeing that assignments are completed and that scheduling is adhered to takes on a unique character under 9,9-oriented leadership. The idea is to make it unnecessary to give frequent or specific directions of the "Now do this; next do that" variety. By getting an understanding among staff members as to what is important to accomplish, and by agreement on how best to achieve these objectives, the direction to take becomes self-evident. The 9,9-oriented nursing administrator's job is to maintain involvement in objectives rather than to rely on obedience of staff members to get work done. She sets little store in formal authority; rather, respect is gained from her skill in aiding staff members to participate in ways that permit them to see the same pathway of what needs to be done as is seen by her.

"I keep informed of progress and influence staff members by identifying problems and, as necessary, by revising goals *with* them. I assist when needed by removing barriers."

Laverne is a 9,9-oriented head nurse. She faces a problem of an over-crowded unit. By involving the staff nurses in taking the necessary action to improve their situation rather than imposing her own solution she gains cooperation in dealing with the problem.

Thus far the morning has gone well for Laverne on 3 West even though two additional surgical patients were transferred from 2 South a couple of hours ago. The staff nurses have been able to handle the extra load with no problem.

At ten o'clock she receives a call from the administrative officer, Lorene Milburn. "Laverne, I'm sending another patient. There are no other beds available."

Laverne mentally checklists her beds and the number of staff nurses on duty. "Give me ten minutes to evaluate our situation, Ms. Milburn. With two cases we received earlier, I'm not sure whether we can handle one more or not."

She hangs up and soon all of the staff nurses are at her station. Lavern reviews her conversation with Lorene Milburn and discusses the alternatives she sees with them. "You may have a better idea," continues Laverne, "but since we will be short one bed with these three new cases, we will have to set up a bed in the hall or tell Ms. Milburn to check out some other possibilities."

"Laverne, I have an idea," Darlene, one of the staff nurses, volunteers. "I think Mrs. Goldman in 216 will share her room. She doesn't need private care anymore. I'll ask her, of course, but I'm positive she'll be agreeable. That way I can handle both of them easily."

"I can help Darlene," says Norma, another staff nurse. "Mr. Ledman checks out tomorrow and the rest of my patients are fairly stable."

"Great," responds Laverne. "Please let me know if you need any help or if problems arise. I'll call Ms. Milburn and tell her everything is set for the admission."

This is a 9,9-oriented team approach in that the head nurse furnishes staff members with information that is important for them to know to do their assignments and to grapple with the changing situation. After giving them the necessary background, she involves them by getting their ideas on what can be done. Commitment on their part comes about as they resolve the problem through open discussion.

Follow-up

The 9,9-oriented nursing administrator follows up or works with her staff in an open and constructive way. In circumstances where a problem exists, she seeks to learn all the facts in the situation and to evaluate the point of view of everyone involved.

"I follow up with those who are responsible. We evaluate how things went and see what we can learn from our experience and how we can apply our learning in the future."

Once staff members have reached a shared basis of understanding and commitment, a 9,9-oriented nursing administrator may find herself having little need to worry about whether a project or assignment has been completed well. With effective leadership, which can arouse *sound* participation, the probability is increased that solutions achieved will be sound and fundamental, not needing constant review and revision.

In the following example, Nelda, a head nurse, and Jill, staff nurse, work toward a common understanding by going over what had happened and agreeing on what might have been done better, and should be done differently the next time around.

Nelda moves quickly down the hall toward room 301 to check on Jill, the new staff nurse. As she enters the room she notices that the patient is in obvious discomfort. Jill is struggling to fit the leg traction properly.

"Here, let me help," offers Nelda and adjusts the weights to a comfortable fit.

Later, out of the patient's hearing, Jill says, slightly flushing, "I'm sorry, Nelda, I couldn't seem to get it right."

"No wonder; you had too much weight." Nelda looks at Jill directly. "Have you ever done this before?"

With downcast eyes Jill replies, "No, actually the situation never arose."

"Well, never mind about that," says Nelda. "I'll go through it and then we'll go to the nurse's station and discuss any other areas you feel uncertain about."

"Thanks, Nelda. I would appreciate that. There *are* a couple of things I'm unsure about." Jill seems relieved at not being scolded, and as they walk back to the station, they are actively discussing Jill's lack of experience in some areas of her job and what to do to help her fill in the gaps.

Nelda's approach to follow-up is 9,9 because she assesses the situation and draws out the facts regarding Jill's lack of experience, but in a way that permits Jill to feel free in accepting help. She then involves Jill in taking next steps.

COMMUNICATION

The 9,9-oriented nursing administrator presents problems in honest, realistic, and objective terms. This means that she describes any given problem in terms of what the current difficulty being encountered is, what is seen to be its cause, and what the consequences of handling this problem in various ways might be.

Stated in reverse, this means that the administrator does not alter the message just to make it easy to swallow. She is factual and applies no sugarcoating. She does not simply pass out the word in a way that leaves people the option of picking it up or not as they wish. Nor does she force the message down staff members' throats as an edict. Neither does she use a public relations approach of trying to make things look more positive than they are.

The nursing administrator may also indicate possible solutions if clearcut ideas are available as to what a good solution might be. The staff comes to understand what the problem is as she sees it. Then if they see it in a different way, they are in an excellent position to get the nursing administrator to recognize, accept, and correct whatever limitations there may have been in her own understanding of the problem. This can be done by pointing out the discrepancies between how the nursing administrator describes the problem and how they understand it.

In the following example, Fran, a head nurse, gets help from her staff in seeking ways to change a new and unsatisfactory policy.

Fran is on her way back to her unit. She thinks about the head nurse meeting she has just left and goes over in her mind again the change in policy regarding paychecks. The new policy is that paychecks will be picked up in the nursing office on Thursday from 9 a.m. to 3 p.m. only. Previously, the night nurses could pick up their paychecks when coming off duty between 7 and 7:30. Fran knows it will create a hardship not only for the night nurses, but also for all those who are off duty Thursday and Friday. The office will not distribute the checks on Saturday and Sunday.

In her mind, the policy is being changed to accommodate a few supervisors who take morning report and then go to coffee. Also, the secretary doesn't settle in until about nine o'clock, so it is to the secretary's convenience to change the hours of picking up the paychecks from 7 a.m. to 9 a.m.

She thinks how she and Elsie had been the only head nurses openly opposed to the rigid rules, asking for reconsideration. She wished Faye Gill, the director of nurses, would have been stronger in resisting the change in hours.

Now Fran is going to her staff with the news about the change in pickup times. From past experience, Fran knows that, because her staff nurses will have objections and frustrations from the change, she will be seeing Ms. Gill with a list of alternatives from her staff whether Ms. Gill likes it or not.

At the staff meeting Fran explains the situation. Reactions are strongly against the change, and several have ideas. Fran draws up a list of methods that could be implemented so that none of the nurses suffer inconvenience in receiving their paychecks. Later she has a meeting with Ms. Gill to go over them.

"I see your group really objects," says Ms. Gill. "I've had complaints from other units, too. It's apparent it was a bad decision that was not thought through too well. Let me keep your list and I'll discuss yours and the other units' complaints with the administrator."

This is a 9,9-oriented approach because Fran enlists the aid of staff members in identifying how the policy will affect them and in developing alternative ways of arranging the paycheck schedule that make sense to everyone. With this approach the head nurse presents the problem and listens to the views of others. Subordinates do not feel that they are being ramrodded, and see that Fran has the ability to influence in their behalf.

The 9,9-oriented nursing administrator strives to get agreement on the real problem and on the best solution as agreed upon by staff members. A 9,9 skill is in helping others express themselves openly and in thinking through options and alternatives so that the best answer emerges. Whether this best answer comes from the nursing administrator or the staff is not important; what is important is that it is identified and used. This means that a premium is placed on her skill in listening.

The 9,9-oriented nursing administrator listens to the staff to understand the ideas they are attempting to sketch in words. She does not listen in order to agree but to gain understanding before commenting. The goal is to get each of these ideas well defined and understood so that issues can be evaluated in the light of logically connected facts. Then when an idea is right it can be used. When it is not, the person who presented it can see its shortcomings in terms of actual evidence. Then the person can abandon it without loss of face.

Communication has an authentic quality among members of a 9,9-oriented nursing team. Openness and honesty in a nursing administrator bring forth similar qualities in the staff. When she is authentic, the staff knows that candor on their part is welcome and put to constructive use. Communication that is 9,9-oriented promotes an "everybody wins" situation because it creates the strongest likelihood that each person's knowledge and skills will be brought into use. This means, too, that team members feel directly involved in the problem's solution. By the very fact of staff participation, the solution becomes genuine and thus earns their full commitment to implementing it.

Under the 9,9 orientation in the following example, Kaye, head nurse, discusses a situation directly with Grace, staff nurse, before it becomes a real problem.

Monday a three-year-old boy, Danny, was admitted to Kaye's unit with problems severe enough to indicate a long hospital stay. The parents are naturally concerned about the welfare of their child.

Kaye notices a tension and aloofness about the young mother whenever Kaye sees her on the unit. Kaye mentions her feelings about the mother to Grace, who is taking care of Danny.

"I never really noticed, Kaye. I guess I've been too busy to be aware of it. I do know she just sits there and refuses to leave when I'm giving him special treatment." Grace goes on to reveal that she feels that many parents inhibit their children's recovery and she feels the less interaction she has with the parents the better.

"You may be right about some parents' worries bothering the child, but in this hospital we feel it is necessary to find out more about what's going on with the mother. Perhaps she needs more information, and the more you ignore her, the more tension she feels. I think you ought to find out what the problem is." Kaye suggests that the next time Danny's mother is at the hospital Grace discuss with her any feelings she might have about the hospital care her child is receiving.

Kaye wanted to ensure, for the child's sake, that negative attitudes were not having a damaging effect. By having a discussion between Grace and the mother, underlying tensions can be revealed and a resolution of them can be brought about.

CONFLICT

Conflict can delay or prevent the achievement of objectives and personal goals. On the other hand, conflict can promote innovation, creativity, and development of new ideas. The 9,9 approach to conflict rests on the assumption that, although conflict is inevitable, it is resolvable. *The key is in how conflict is managed.* The best approach to conflict is to anticipate it and to take steps to ensure understanding and agreement before staff members take polarized positions. This is not always possible. When conflict does arise, confrontation to diagnose the causes and to find the optimal way of handling it is the 9,9-oriented approach. There are two distinct meanings in the way that the word *confrontation* is used, and because there is no good substitute for this term, it is important to distinguish between them.

Confrontation-as-combat

One meaning of confrontation is "beyond contest but falling short of actual combat." It rests upon the concept of bringing opposing points of view into sharp focus. This meaning of confrontation is motivated by a wish to test one's strength against that of another. The underlying assumption is that one view or person will prevail over the other.

Confrontation-as-comparison

Confrontation-as-comparison, a quite different meaning of confrontation, involves bringing opposing points of view into the same sharp focus, but with the aim of resolving differences based on understanding and agreement. There is no commitment to the idea that one point of view should prevail. The result may be that one point of view does prevail. If this occurs, it is because the other person has learned that there are necessary and sufficient reasons for accepting one position and rejecting the other. It may be that neither point of view prevails. Out of the comparison and contrast, an emergent position is identified.

Viewed by an observer, *confrontation-as-combat* and *confrontation-as-comparison* might appear similar. An important underlying difference makes the distinction clear. In confrontation-as-combat there is a contest of will; the holder of one point of view feels threatened by the holder of the other. Yielding means accepting a resolution based on weakness. No one wants to lose.

Confrontation-as-comparison takes place when trust exists among those who are trying to resolve the difference. Trust implies goodwill and good intentions. To win is unimportant; to find a sound solution is all-important. Under these conditions, one person yielding to the position of another is not capitulation. It entails no loss of face. It is not a measure of weakness. Rather, it is the opposite—a demonstration of commitment to a best solution premised on the use of logic and reason and an understanding of emotions.

Confrontation-as-combat is related to the kind of win-lose power struggle that frequently occurs when one or both protagonists have a 9,1 orientation, that is, "*Who* is right?" Confrontation-as-comparison is motivated by an orientation toward 9,9 fulfillment through contribution, that is, "*What* is right?"

How might a 9,9-oriented nursing administrator deal with what appears to be an irreconcilable conflict? Two talented members submit mutually exclusive recommendations that will provide a basis for needed coordination within the department. The 9,1-oriented boss might accept the recommendation she believes easiest to implement and veto the other. This approach produces a win-lose situation between the staff members. Wishing to avoid this adverse effect, the nursing administrator might decide to take a 5,5-oriented action to compromise the difference, taking something from both recommendations and putting them together, even though the final product will not be as good as one of the two initially proposed. Or, this nursing administrator might accept both staff member's recommendations but then procrastinate in a 1,1 way, hoping to avoid the need for decisiveness. Any of these alternatives may cause coordination to break down and antagonisms and resentment to be felt. Or both staff members may feel dissatisfied and poorly motivated to make the solution work or frustrated at the nursing administrator's inaction. Which approach the nursing administrator takes depends on her concept of what is likely to be most "effective"—a subjective choice.

What appears as flexibility to a situationally oriented supervisor is likely to be experienced by colleagues and subordinates as shifty, untrustworthy, even deceitful, whether or not dishonesty is involved or intended. The unpredictable aspect provokes suspicion, distrust, closedness, hiding, resentment, antagonism, or calculation and tactics, depending on the Grid orientations of the colleague or subordinate who experiences it.

The 9,9-oriented nursing administrator who has the capacity for versatility might do something else to resolve the coordination problem. She might bring the staff members together to face the contradictory character of their recommendations and help them find a way to work together to solve their problems. Shared points of view, previously unrecognized, begin to emerge. As areas of similarity appear and differences are pared down, agreements essential for coordinated effort are realized. Mutual respect is maintained throughout, with confidence that the solution ultimately reached is more likely to be valid and easier to implement.

If this approach does not work as anticipated, it might be necessary for a 9,9-oriented nursing administrator to shift tactics. The alternative might now involve the staff members cooperating in designing and running an experiment to test the operational consequences of both approaches, or in putting aside their introductory proposals and formulating an "ideal" solution. Each of these different approaches is still based on 9,9 assumptions.

Mistakes and errors

The 9,9-oriented approach to mistakes and errors relies on good teamwork. Because 9,9-oriented team colleagues feel responsibility for one another, they can be expected to help anyone who is having difficulty. A nursing administrator realizes that there are at least three general causes of mistakes and errors. The first is whenever the staff does not have necessary technical skills or background to carry out tasks. When a mistake occurs because of lack of skill, a 9,9 approach in the short term is on-the-job coaching.

A second cause of mistakes and errors arises at the planning stage when there is inadequate understanding of those involved. The administrator may have glossed over points that the staff *thinks* they understand but actually do not. Perhaps she fails to recognize either the staff's need to probe more deeply into a problem or their hidden reservations and doubts.

If a nursing administrator is 9,9-oriented, she may recognize a third source as an additional factor. A point to check is whether a staff member is being turned off by a job that poses less challenge and success through accomplishment than the staff member feels capable of achieving. Boredom can be a factor in causing mistakes and errors. When this happens, the 9,9-oriented nursing administrator meets with the staff member and works toward redesigning activities and responsibilities. In this way, the challenge the job contains can be increased by making it more varied or more responsible and in these ways putting new interest into it. This is work enrichment. It is not a cosmetic face lift of an enlarged collection of boring chores, but a development avenue for the individual who wants to contribute further to the hospital and to patient care.

A 9,9-oriented nursing administrator's reaction to a staff member's mistake can be summed up in this way:

"I understand you have made a mistake. Let's review the details of what happened. We can figure out what brought it about and then take steps to correct it and to establish procedures so that it doesn't happen again."

In the following example, Jane, a head nurse, confronts Lucille and later Beth, both staff nurses, with a mistake that had proven costly.

There is a memo on Jane's desk this morning with a copy of the hospital budget attached. There is a large red asterisk beside "catheterization sets" with a note from the nursing administrator asking her to find out why the number of sets greatly increased last month. Upon checking, Jane narrows it down to orders beginning the week of her vacation two weeks ago.

She meets with Lucille, who covered for her during that time. She explains the situation.

"Beth had just come on our unit at that time, as you remember. No one had ever told her about the setup and she kept contaminating the sets. She had never asked either. And I was so busy that week I guess I didn't follow up with her as close as I should have."

"Well, I goofed in not having a checklist for orientees," Jane replies. "One thing we can do is to talk with Beth and make sure she understands all our procedures as of now. Another is for you and me to develop a checklist for orienting new employees."

This is a 9,9-oriented approach because Jane seeks out the details of what happened and follows up with the persons involved to prevent the mistake from happening again. Both Jane and Lucille come to realize their shortcomings. Beth will benefit, too, because she may have unresolved reservations and doubts that could result in mistakes in the future. Once her problems are worked through she will be able to give her full commitment to an agreed-upon way of doing things.

Complaints

Complaints are viewed by the 9,9-oriented nursing administrator as signals of real or potential problems that need attention. Expression of negative feelings offers her the opportunity to deal with people on issues that are bothering them.

Dealing with complaints is essentially a question of identifying the *real* problem. To illustrate, recall that all staff members who can contribute are present at a scheduled conference. This makes for a different situation than when individual staff members come to the nursing administrator one by one to voice a complaint privately. When a staff member comes to her to voice a complaint and only the two are present, there is seldom any immediate access to evidence outside the person. In the team situation, a nursing administrator has more sources of information to draw on when complaint issues are raised. Most issues are not so personal that privacy is required. Furthermore, each person learns something by public discussion, and professional standards are likely to be strengthened. Granted that openness can be overdone and abused, the 9,9-oriented nursing administrator is careful to recognize when a complaint is truly private.

A 9,9-oriented nursing administrator's attitude about complaints can be summed up in this way:

"When you have a complaint, let's discuss it, analyze it, and, if other parties are involved, we'll include them also. That way we can resolve it quickly, more likely to everyone's satisfaction."

Given her high concern for staff members, the 9,9-oriented nursing administrator does not consider nor accept as private a complaint that involves other team members. She will say, "Look, there may be a problem here that is better put on the table where everyone can take a look at it. Will you agree then, Phyllis, to bring this up at a meeting I will convene as early as possible?" This is already testing the *reality* of Phyllis's complaint. When Phyllis brings it up in the meeting there is a greater likelihood that the problem will be viewed from more angles, and with greater objectivity than when a complaint is dealt with privately on a one-to-one basis.

The *real* problem for a 9,9-oriented nursing administrator may or may not be the particular words a staff member is using to complain, but some part of it certainly has to do with personal feelings. One step in identifying the problem is to help this person bring out her emotions. Those that are caused by existing problems of communication can be remedied by providing needed information. Complaints that arise from malfunction of equipment can be easily resolved. Complaints that are personal are another story, as mentioned previously.

In summary, the 9,9-oriented nursing administrator does not treat a complaint as just inevitable bitching or as something to be soothed, ignored, or put aside for a cooling-off period. The complaint is a reality because it means that one or more of the staff are concerned about something they see as being wrong. The nursing administrator first draws out the facts that caused the underlying feelings, involving all staff members.

In the following example, Jo, head nurse, challenges her staff nurse, Cindy, who is complaining about the lack of cooperation by other nurses with Mr. Frazier, a patient. Cindy is asking them to consider a different perspective on how to handle him.

Cindy West, a staff nurse, meets Jo in the hall and says, "Mr. Frazier in room 14B is giving me a fit. He's a real sorehead. Nothing suits him. The LPN and aides will answer all other patients' lights to help me out, but they refuse to answer his because of his constant complaining. I can't be everywhere at once, and they are not carrying their load. I suppose he's going to want to see you about the care he's getting here."

Jo asks, "Does he mention anything specifically?"

"No," says Cindy. "It seems to me it's everything. Besides, Dr. Jenson saw him this morning and I think he told Mr. Frazier about having to go to surgery again."

"Okay," says Jo. "I'll go in and see what I can do."

Jo talks to Mr. Frazier who admits that he feels neglected because the nurses don't come when he rings. He is lonesome and would like someone to talk to. He doesn't like the hospital food. She also finds out that because of family problems his wife cannot visit him. The prospect of having to face additional surgery has left him in a depleted emotional state.

Later Jo meets with her staff. Several voice their own complaints about Mr. Frazier. Jo shares with them what she has learned about Mr. Frazier so that everyone has a clearer understanding of his situation. Several suggestions are made that can ease his frustration.

Jo not only brings out into the open the feelings of Mr. Frazier and staff nurses, she also sheds new light on "why" Mr. Frazier is being difficult. This results in specific actions to be taken to deal with his complaints.

Hostile feelings

The 9,9-oriented nursing administrator knows that tensions that might expand into hostile feelings should be resolved whenever they arise so that they have little opportunity to build up. The concept is that hostile feelings are important because they exist, and therefore need to be dealt with in a sound manner. If the nursing administrator is alert to those aspects of behavior that support a 9,9 orientation, her relationship with the staff can be strengthened, with two main benefits resulting. One is better productivity. The other is that staff members are ready to participate more actively and to give their involvement and commitment. Listening to what a staff member says invites a staff member to listen to what the nursing administrator says. Being open invites openness; reacting without defensiveness invites nondefensive responses.

The nursing administrator's attitude is:

"I am open to discussing hostile emotions. If we can talk about why you feel as you do, then we will have made a start in finding out what the real problem is."

In the following situation, Margaret, a head nurse, calmly and openly listens to Lisa's grievance against her.

Margaret had not been on 2 East long before she detected hostility toward her by Lisa, staff nurse. It was also evident in Lisa's attitude toward other staff members, and even the patients. There were a couple of times when Margaret had walked into a patient's room and overheard Lisa being unnecessarily curt with the patient.

One day Margaret confronts Lisa about her attitude toward everyone. "Lisa, since I have been on this floor, I have felt that you resent me. I am wondering if this has anything to do with your attitude toward your patients."

At first Lisa seemed hesitant to express herself. She keeps her eyes down for a few minutes and then, seemingly relieved for an opportunity to get it out, blurts out, "I wanted your job very badly and felt I deserved it. When they passed over me I felt very dejected."

"I can imagine you did," responded Margaret. "Do you know *why* you weren't considered?"

"It was my fault, actually." Lisa slightly blushes as she goes on. "I never went to the director of nurses to ask her if I could have the job. I just felt that they would pick me because I have been here the longest. So I guess there's really no one for me to blame but myself."

"If you are really serious about moving ahead, Lisa, why don't you discuss it with the director? She will know you are interested, and then if an opportunity arises, you'll be ready for it."

"You're right. I guess I wanted to be handed something rather than initiating any effort."

This handling of Lisa's reaction is in the 9,9 orientation. Margaret confronts Lisa to find out what the real problem is. But she does not stop there. Lisa was also able to see that her own lack of initiative was the cause of her feeling the way she did and of her curt behavior with others.

A 9,9-oriented nursing administrator recognizes that hostile feelings are symptomatic that something is not okay. This does not mean that she sees the staff members as "bad" or "no good" because she has these feelings. The first desire is to know what it is that is producing these reactions. This means that she communicates to the staff members that she really wants to understand the causes behind the friction. It means that the staff member can talk freely without the nursing administrator becoming judgmental at the first negative thing that is said.

DEVELOPMENT

The orientation and development of a new staff member is sometimes a complicated process. An example of an effective approach is when the nursing administrator meets regularly with the new staff member to review her experiences and formulate with the staff member her own training needs.

During the initial orientation, the chief issue is in the staff member having the information necessary for measuring her chances of being able to contribute effectively to the hospital organization in a personally rewarding way. This means that the nursing administrator provides a realistic assessment of the hospital's strengths and weaknesses, promotion practices, and the like. She avoids holding out unrealistic promises and hopes.

"I try to see that work requirements are matched with the staff member's capabilities or needs for development in making decisions as to who does what."

In the following example, Loretta, head nurse, is discussing with Jeannette, a new staff nurse, the plans for her employment on 5 South.

"One of the first things we will do," Loretta is saying, "is to assign you a nurse to help you learn the routine here. The in-service department also has several programs coming up that I think will be good for you to attend. By the way, how did things go this morning in your discussion with Ms. Graden about pay and fringe benefits?"

"Just fine," replies Jeannette. "I may have some questions later, but everything is clear right now."

"After you have been here a couple of weeks," Loretta continues, "we'll discuss your feelings about how we do things and go over any problems you might have. As time goes by we will do some future planning as to what further development you might need."

This is a 9,9-oriented approach because Loretta has a high concern for seeing that Jeannette is brought on board in a satisfactory manner. She also plans for future steps for development of goals that will improve Jeannette's performance on the unit, as well as establishes a time period to discuss Jeannette's reactions to her orientation.

The key to performance evaluation under 9,9 lies in the concept of *goal setting*. The review setting offers an opportunity for the nursing administrator and staff member jointly to discuss the present level of performance and to plot a future pathway toward eliminating barriers and toward achieving mutually agreed upon goals. Barriers to the staff nurse's development are identified, and may range all the way from technical considerations to highly personal ones. These also may include aspects of the nursing administrator's behavior and other features of the work setting, as well as factors over which the staff nurse herself has direct control. These can be alleviated only through action in the helper sense as described earlier.

Although evaluation is not absent, it is not seen as the sole responsibility of the nursing administrator to judge the actions of the staff nurse. Thus, the evaluation situation is extended far beyond assessment of past performance, to include diagnosing, planning, and follow-up for change.

In the following example, Shirley, head nurse, conducts a 9,9-oriented performance appraisal with Noreen, staff nurse. Shirley is well prepared and builds on a solid relationship, which is one of easy, two-way give and take.

Shirley is contemplating the scheduled annual evaluation that is to take place today with Noreen. She discussed this with Noreen two weeks ago and they had chosen this particular date on which to review Noreen's past year's performance.

Shirley is well prepared for the interview. She is confident not only about the accuracy of her reactions but also of her and Noreen's well-established and shared knowledge of the grounds on which these evaluations are to be made. During the past year they had talked about her performance five or six times. At one point Shirley had told her, citing the evidence, that she still seemed unsure of herself in her relationships with the patients and doctors. Another time Noreen had panicked in an emergency situation. Shirley discussed both these situations with Noreen and they had agreed upon improvement goals they both felt to be attainable. Since then, Noreen has made substantial progress, particularly on her uncertainty. Shirley is now able to point out that the doctors have commented on her more relaxed attitudes. Shirley had set up on-the-job emergency simulations to help Noreen overcome her feeling of helplessness in the emergency, and both feel that real progress has been made.

Noreen studies Shirley's report for several minutes and then says, "Shirley, I'm satisfied with the report. I know I've made progress. I feel good about it. In a few additional areas I'm not satisfied with how I do things, and I am going to try to improve in each of them. Now, here are improvements I think can be made. I will need your help on some of them."

They discuss the list Noreen has developed. Shirley is impressed with her suggestions, and they quickly begin to think in concrete terms as to what each can do to help Noreen move forward.

INTRODUCTION OF CHANGE

A 9,9-oriented director of nurses or head nurse introduces changes only after their ramifications have been weighed. She seeks to know all the facts of the situation, carefully weighing the pros and cons, and then meets with her staff to gain the benefit of their ideas.

In the following example, Linda Blackstone meets with the head nurses to discuss the unit manager issue.

Linda Blackstone, director of nursing, is conducting a meeting with the head nurses. They are discussing a proposed plan for hiring a unit manager for the units. Each head nurse already has expressed her opinion as to what the change will mean to her personally. A few express reservations about some of their "favorite duties" being given up, and others express relief at the prospect of having assistance with administrative details. They all agree, however, that a change is needed because something must be done to alleviate the administrative paperwork in this hospital.

"I don't know," says Glenda, one of the head nurses, "personally I think a unit manager will be more of a hindrance than a help."

Linda responds, "That could be true, Glenda. But on the other hand, I know that you have really been burdened down with a lot of paperwork the last several months and it's beginning to tell."

"Yes, I guess you're right. I have certainly been overloaded," Glenda responds, adding, "a unit manager may help, and I'm prepared to give it a real chance to succeed. When will this take place?"

Under the 9,9 orientation, Linda makes sure that doubts are aired so that the change is one to which everyone is committed. She views change as an option that provides a better way of doing things, and Glenda comes to this point of view. Both are prepared to make it successful, and Linda is willing to try.

REACTIONS TO 9,9 SUPERVISION

Many people have never had real experience with 9,9 ways of supervising and are not in a position to evaluate it in comparison to their more negative past experiences. They may have learned to regard a 9,9 orientation as unrealistic from earlier experiences and from the currently existing culture of their hospital. To be in a position to evaluate 9,9 teamwork, nursing administrators need to learn the skills essential for exercising this kind of supervision.

A 9,9 way of involving people in getting results is consistent with sound behavioral science principles as applied to supervision. For this reason, staff members might be expected to react to this approach to supervision with enthusiasm. Most do. However, this is not always the case.

Can-do spirit

One of the most common reactions to the 9,9 approach is positive readiness to be involved and to make the commitments necessary for achieving the kind of excellence that 9,9 teamwork makes possible. This reaction results because many staff nurses strive for a greater degree of involvement than has been possible for them under other styles of nursing administrator behavior. Striving to achieve goals in which the nursing administrator has personal investment presents a challenge and results in staff members having a stake in seeing their particular unit in the hospital succeed.

It's too much to ask

Another reaction acknowledges that 9,9 teamwork is a realistic possibility, but claims it expects too much of a staff person. The requirements of involvement, participation, and commitment are beyond what many staff nurses are ready to consider for themselves. Others might have been ready to make such commitments earlier in their employment yet have pulled back and taken their commitments elsewhere—into the community, into hobbies, into service agencies, and so on. This is understandable because to make the effort that a 9,9 approach involves might upset a staff member's current status quo. Without experiencing the alternative, maintaining the status quo may seem preferable to her.

It's impractical

Another reaction is "It's impractical; it takes too much time. It won't work. My superior manage that way? Never!" Many staff people have become so conditioned by their past supervisory experiences under certain nursing administrators that they can dismiss the 9,9 teamwork idea as hypothetical and impractical in the sense of being too ideal to be realized. They have seen too much of what really goes on in terms of other Grid approaches to supervision to believe that the values inherent in 9,9 might ever be embraced throughout a hospital. Therefore, the attitude is that 9,9 ideas are unrealistic.

Embracing 9,9 values is not the same as acquiring the skills essential for bringing 9,9 teamwork into everyday use. A learning phase is essential for bringing a 9,9 basis of teamwork into operation. The kind of learning involved requires more than simply reading a book, seeing a movie, or answering questions. Strategies for learning 9,9 techniques are discussed in Chapter 9.

SUMMARY

The 9,9 orientation is based on a shared sense of involvement, participation, and commitment. It calls for a different kind of nursing administrator–staff member interaction than is found in other Grid styles.

Under the 9,9 approach, planning and scheduling is done with the involvement of the staff. The nursing administrator, with them, establishes schedules, ground rules, and procedures and sets up individual responsibilities. Direction is not given on a task-by-task basis except under unique emergency or last-resort circumstances. Work assignments are carried out based on shared understanding and agreement; therefore staff members operate on a more or less self-regulated basis.

Follow-up with staff members is important. A 9,9-oriented nursing administrator seeks to involve her staff in critiquing themselves and in teamwork in order for them to learn from experience.

Communication is an open, candid, and free exchange between the nursing administrator and staff member. Neither needs to be on guard in order to avoid misunderstanding by the other.

Mistakes and errors are viewed as being caused by deficiencies in the learning background that must be rectified in order to avoid or reduce them in the future. This view rejects ideas of blame or punishment and looks toward corrective actions that eliminate causes.

Complaints may arise from any number of sources, but the important point in 9,9-oriented supervision is that complaints be accepted at face value, be understood, dealt with, and solved. This can be done by diagnosing the complaint prior to trying to "answer" it. Often the stated complaint is not the real problem, and only by getting beneath the surface can the difficulty be resolved.

A 9,9-oriented nursing administrator views hostile feelings as indicative of real problems in the work situation. Such emotions are danger signals and they are reacted to in a very serious-minded way. Open, candid, authentic interaction with the subordinate under nonjudgmental, nondefensive conditions permits genuine interaction of the kind essential for understanding them and for taking corrective actions to eliminate causes responsible for hostile feelings.

Development that is 9,9-oriented relates performance to previously set goals and objectives. In this way, performance evaluation takes place on an objective, operational, problem-solving level. It then becomes possible for the nursing administrator to help staff members see what has caused an excellent level to be reached, surpassed, or missed, by whatever margin. When objectives are set realistically high and have been met, nursing excellence is the result.

Change is introduced only after the ramifications of a proposal have been carefully evaluated. The nursing administrator seeks out all the facts carefully, weighing the pros and cons in her own mind, and then meets with staff and others whom any damage would affect to gain the benefit of their reactions and ideas before changes are implemented.

Chapter 8

COMBINATIONS OF GRID THEORIES

Additional orientations can be identified beyond the five basic ones already described. These are combinations of the "pure" theories. They involve the coupling of two or more of the basic approaches already discussed—9,9; 5,5; 9,1; 1,9; or 1,1—being used as an administrative approach. The three to be focused on include maternalism (paternalism), the two-hat approach, and the statistical 5,5 orientation.

MATERNALISM

Maternalism denotes a relationship between an administrative nurse and staff members that involves a 9,1-oriented kind of concern for production coupled with 1,9-motivated approval-giving. This is similar to what sometimes happens between a parent and a child when compliance is expected by the parent, who gives love and approval in acknowledgement of obedience. A maternalistic administrative nurse retains tight control in work matters, telling staff nurses in no uncertain terms who, what, where, and how (but often not why). Yet this person is generous, kind, and supporting in a personal way when subordinates do what they have been told.

The spirit of maternalism is seen when an administrative nurse calls a staff member over about an hour before the end of the shift and says, "Helen, you've put in a good day's work and finished all your assignments early. Why don't we go and have a cup of coffee and a cigarette in the nurse's lounge?" Gratitude for compliance is expressed through personal warmth and thoughtfulness.

A maternalistic nurse treats staff members as part of the agency family by telling them how to perform every activity. She encourages them to be responsible, but they are likely to avoid exercising initiative because the administrative nurse is unable to delegate. She constantly checks whenever someone seems involved with a problem not previously discussed. Staff members soon learn that she is never happy with them unless they are handling it precisely as she would have had them deal with it had they come for advice in the first place.

The result of this way of administering becomes painfully clear when the

105

supervisor is heard to describe staff members in this way: "My staff won't accept responsibility. They are bright and capable, with plenty of know-how, but they check everything with me first. They won't take the ball and run. It is difficult to see how they will ever succeed." What she fails to realize is that staff nurses want to please her and yet they feel the need for double-checking because she promotes a sense of uncertainty that undercuts the confidence necessary for them to act autonomously.

Maternalism can become so widely practiced that it pervades the hospital. The reward for compliance with a maternalist's wish to be "mother" is economic and social security; thus staff members prefer being dependent for guidance to acting on their own. Those who buckle under are given many fine things from top administration—good pay, excellent benefit programs, recreational facilities, retirement programs, to say nothing of personal acceptance and feelings of security. These welfare items, in exchange for compliance and dependency, do tend to increase the workers' sense of well-being. "I owe my soul to the company store," is a line from a famous song about feelings toward paternalistic administration once a person has become so locked in that there is no escape.

The maternalistic nursing administrator controls some of these benefits through the evaluation system. If the staff member does not comply, there may not be a recommendation for increases or other benefits.

A director of nurses who has fought for pay increases and benefits cannot understand it when the staff makes further demands. This time it is for bettering working conditions. The director of nurses responds by saying, "I've given them all these good things but they are never satisfied." The staff may even begin to negotiate with the union.

With consistent applications over time, maternalism can create a highly stable organization, with minimum turnover, as hospital agency members obey requirements placed on them in exchange for material security. However, some of the worst upheavals and disruptions have occurred where maternalism has become extensively practiced. Against a background of what appears to be a stable and long-enduring agency, waves of resentment and retaliation have broken out against the management that has for so long treated its people so well. Such a gross shift from compliant acceptance to defiant retaliation appears contradictory.

One way of understanding these reactions is this: 9,1-oriented supervision of work rejects and disregards the thinking and capabilities of people. This generates frustration and resistance as well as produces feelings of alienation. These feelings are difficult or impossible to express directly toward an employer who, at the same time, offers economic, social, and personal security to those who comply with unilateral demands. Reactions to indignities, as a result, may be swallowed and bottled up, but they are still there. By masking that seething resentment and unrest, the appearance of docility, devotion, and loyalty is produced. Under these circumstances, however, even a minor irritation can serve as a trigger that causes an eruption of vitriolic and hateful reactions. *The formula for concocting hate consists of arousing frustrations under conditions of dependence.* The reason is that one feels antagonized and aggressive but cannot fight back because of one's fear of losing acceptance and security. Although maternalism has failed repeatedly to solve problems of getting production through people, it is still a rather widespread attitude underlying much supervisory thinking. There are many variations on maternalism which look different but actually differ from one another only in terms of degree. The benevolent autocrat is another way of saying maternalist, and "missionary" is another variation on the same style.

TWO-HAT APPROACH

Using the two-hat approach, a nursing administrator practices 9,1-oriented supervision in daily work but removes her production hat at six-month or yearly intervals and puts on a 1,9-oriented "people" hat to counsel with staff nurses in ways that deal mainly with attitudes at large and only incidentally with real issues that relate to work effectiveness. Under the two-hat approach, performance appraisal is not part and parcel of work activity and professional development. Rather, it is a scheduled activity and is concentrated on only when the "people" hat is worn. Head nurses are likely to view this kind of performance discussion as an activity they must engage in, not because it contributes to improved work and development, but because the nursing office has placed them under obligation to conduct these sessions as a matter of organization policy.

The two-hat approach also can be seen as an organization-wide practice. For example, on one day, say Monday, the director of nurses meets with her staff and discusses problems and inefficient operations. Then on another day, say Wednesday, the same group meets again. This time they discuss people problems, morale issues, and turnover. The actions taken on Monday are intended to solve production problems. They are considered mainly in terms of technical production aspects. Even though they may be tied in with personal problems, they are not likely to be considered in light of their effects on head nurses. The same is true on Wednesday. The people problems considered at that time may include time off and scheduling. They may bear significantly on production, but they are viewed mainly in the light of personal needs. On Monday, problems concerning people are set aside until Wednesday. On Wednesday, production problems are delayed for discussion until the next Monday.

The two concerns are separate but equal in importance. The basic assumption is that though there are two sets of problems there are no inherent connections between them.

The "separate but equal" way of seeing problems is very widespread in our society, and is widely relied upon because at a certain level it "makes sense." You have to simplify things and reduce them in order to grapple with them. If you try to discuss everything at once, that is, how people attitudes impact on production and how production creates people attitudes, it gets hopelessly complicated. Yet it is quickly recognized that both are equally important. It is just that they are different. Therefore, to split them up and deal with them one at a time is a natural way of trying to grapple with problems that seem too complicated to be dealt with as interlaced issues.

Nursing administrators often do the same when asked to evaluate the talents of two staff nurses. Rather than make a comparison and identify the reasons for the promotion of one relative to the other, or the reasons for a merit raise to one relative to the other, the administrator will plead that both nurses are equal, though different. Their competence is essentially the same, but each has a different set of unique skills that make one different from the other while comparable in overall output. What in fact is involved is that the nursing administrator is avoiding the unattractive prospect of making a judgment that might result in drawing criticism, or, if the two staff nurses being evaluated were to learn of her evaluation, one might feel offended and resentful at having been regarded less favorably than the other. The "equal but different" mentality permits the problem to be resolved in such a manner as to avoid real-life comparisons. This approach fails to appreciate that, by taking a broader perspective, the strengths and weaknesses of several persons can be identified and evaluated and generalizations drawn that permit unequalness to be seen, even when certain uniqueness or differences between them are present.

Of course, drawing distinctions between people is only pertinent in administrative work when decisions for promotion, merit raise, development, or discharge are involved in the conclusions being reached. Otherwise it is unnecessary to draw distinctions, and when such distinctions are unnecessary, they are useless.

"STATISTICAL 5,5"

It is occasionally said of an administrative nurse, whether director, head, or charge, "It's hard to tell anything exactly about her leadership style. She fits every position on the Grid at one time or another." The statistical 5,5-oriented nursing administrator employs any two, and sometimes all five, basic styles in dealing with production-people dilemmas. The essential feature is that she manages according to what is thought effective at any particular time. Effectiveness is defined as behavior that is appropriate to the demands of the particular situation. This is an administrative orientation that ignores behavioral science principles.

The reason is that the administrator adjusts to every situation in the way she privately prefers, not in the best or soundest way. For example, if a staff member has no motivation or initiative, the nursing administrator does not assign her important work. Rather she ignores her in a 1,1-oriented way. If a subordinate is easily upset, the supervisor eases up on pressure and praises her, even though rewards may not be justified, using a 1,9-oriented approach. If another staff member is falling behind and is not aware of the impending loss of valued membership, a statistical 5,5-oriented nursing administrator points out that she is failing to carry a fair share of the load and that, unless she does, others will be critical and rejecting. Here the nursing administrator relies on a 5,5 approach. If a staff member has high standards and is being productive, even though this may be producing conflict with others, the nursing administrator spurs her to greater effort to resolve the conflict in a way that maintains production, thus relying on a 9,9-oriented approach. If instructions are arbitrarily resisted by still another staff member, she demands compliance in a 9,1-oriented manner.

The statistical 5,5-oriented head nurse hopscotches all over the Grid, behaving inconsistently by treating each staff member differently, depending upon the staff member. Yet the nursing administrator sees little or no contradiction in these actions. She assumes that each person is different and unique; therefore, creating shared relationships with all the staff members based on mutual dignity and respect simply is not practical. Lacking a concept of change or development, she "maneuvers," trying to adjust the supervision provided to whatever is expected within the boundaries of the status quo.

Most hospitals have no one consistent organization style. Each department or division is left to its own resources without a systematic plan for strengthening supervisory practices. In a more-or-less evolutionary way, these departments and divisions develop their own particular style. One nursing unit may be run as a tight ship to satisfy its 9,1-oriented head nurse, another may do just enough to meet requirements, while a third may strive for excellence. The statistical 5,5 quality in the final analysis is most probably brought about by a hands-off attitude from the top in an organization practicing the policy of extreme decentralization.

Still another aspect of 5,5 statistical behavior is related to the issue, "There is no one best way to solve administrative problems."

The option to "no one best way" is, "How you deal with a problem is contingent on the situation, that is, 'It all depends.'" Many people prefer the "It all depends" answer, and we need to understand why this is so, when in fact there does seem to be one best way, that is, the 9,9 approach, though how it is applied varies with the situation.

Rejection of "one best way" is equivalent to repudiating the proposition that effective behavior is based on scientific principles or laws. Yet the view that principles of behavior undergird specific events is consistent with all other areas of scientific inquiry. We know that principles of physics underlie a vast range of phenomena in inanimate nature. Principles of biology account for phenomena of life and make them predictable. By analogy, behavioral science principles, as described in the 9,9-oriented style in Chapter 7, underlie human conduct, provide guidelines for soundness, and make behavior predictable.

These principles characterize sound behavior, just as there are principles of physics that undergird sound engineering. Violate principles of physics in the engineering of a bridge or a building, for example, and you get disaster. Another example is from the standpoint of nutrition. Nutritionally speaking, there is one best way of maintaining the body in a healthy condition. The strategy involves adhering to nutritional principles as they relate to the intake of protein, fat, and carbohydrates, plus a number of minerals, vitamins, and so on. Not all of the details have been worked out but the principles are well established: intake above an optimum produces obesity; intake beneath the optimum leads to fatigue, malnutrition, weakness, and susceptibility to a number of diseases.

Thus optimum intake is a matter of principle. Disregard it and health troubles are imminent. However, the manner in which the ingredients of sound nutritional behavior are acquired is a tactical matter, contingent upon the availability of various foods. For instance, protein may be acquired from a number of sources. It makes no difference from the standpoint of nutritional principles what the particular source is, but simply that certain substances are acquired. To repudiate the one-best-way idea under the premise that the most effective leadership style "depends upon the situation at any given time," one would have to reject these basic behavioral science propositions.

REJECTION AND REBUTTAL

Contingency theorists reject the concept of one best style of leadership on the basis of at least the following four criteria: no time, no competence, no need, no flexibility.

No time

It is often said that many situations involve crises where there is no time to consult or to share problem solving in a participative way. This usually is interpreted to mean that the supervisor should proceed in a 9,1-oriented manner if acting according to the requirements of the situation. There are two answers to this reason for rejecting a 9,9 orientation. One is that most crises can be avoided or their impact reduced through anticipation. Simulations permit participants to learn to take responsible action in a self-directing way in order to avert tragedy at the time of crisis. This is a 9,9-oriented action, not a 9,1 approach. However, some crises offer no opportunity for anticipation; they just happen. In this case, the supervisor can exercise unilateral judgments to provide order and direction for others. Such action is not "arbitrary," but rather in itself is of a 9,9 character. The administrator is exercising judgment on behalf of others, who, by virtue of the circumstances, are less capable of exercising self-direction.

No competence

Another basis of rejection of the 9,9 approach to nursing administration says that staff members may not be competent to participate. Therefore, it is necessary to tell them what to do in a maternalistic, 9,1-oriented manner or to let them learn from their own errors in the school of hard knocks, which is the equivalent of 1,1 abdication. The 9,9 solution is to help staff members to develop the competence essential for effective participation in problem solving, decision making, and implementation. When this happens, the opportunity for involving others and gaining their thinking and commitment in a 9,9 way replaces the need for 9,1-oriented supervision.

No need

A third criticism is that there are circumstances in which the involvement of staff members would be wasteful because they have no stake in the situation and nothing to contribute. This criticism disregards basic concepts intrinsic to the 9,9 approach, which provides guidelines for when an administrator should act alone, with one staff member or several, or with all in concert, depending on the problem being dealt with. This is not shifting from one Grid style to another, and it does not mean that everybody acts together all the time.

No flexibility

The fourth consideration presumes that a 9,9 action is mechanically the same regardless of the situation. This criticism fails to take into account how the concept of versatility provides a basis for understanding that 9,9 leadership is based consistently on sound principles of behavior used in creative and constructive ways that are (1) unique to particular situations, (2) unlikely to generate negative side effects, (3) optimal for problem solving and productivity, and (4) stimulating to growth and development toward maturity for those in the situation. Relying on behavioral science principles and implementing them through versatile applications is analogous to the relationship between scientific principles in physics and their application to engineering problems. Principles are not violated and disregarded; what changes is the tactics used. Tactics vary depending on the situation.

Compare the different styles of leadership, for example, in the same situation. As part of a new agency start-up, the nursing administrator may start with a group of individuals who have never known or worked with one another. The task is to get the agency on-stream. A situational leadership might provide very close 9,1-oriented management if she assumes that even experienced staff members do not know what to do. When they comply with her directions, she may then give them recognition. If they begin to buck, she might shift to a 1,9 sweetness-and-light approach of encouragement and support, or turn to 1,1-oriented laissez-faire leadership to reduce their antagonisms.

A nursing administrator whose supervision is governed by 9,9-oriented principles of behavior knows, however, that sound results are most likely when she and staff members work as a team to achieve objectives. They can learn to analyze problems. And, even though there are no tried-and-true answers, they seek "best" solutions by confronting differences, relieving disagreements by gathering additional data, simulating a proposal before implementing it, and so on. Beyond that, leadership may involve frequent critique to stimulate operational as well as interpersonal learning.

Principles of behavior in the preceding situation rely on trust and respect. The engineering specifics include mutual goal setting, openness, resolution of disagreements and conflict based on understanding and agreement, learning to change through use of critique, and so forth. These aspects of behavior and performance are verified in social psychology, mental health research, and clinical psychiatry as essential for a sound problem-solving relationship.

GRID SALAD

Self-deception, perceptual distortions, contingency concepts, and statistical 5,5 distortions of a 9,9 orientation all are examples of Grid salad.

It is important for the reader to be aware of Grid salad and to constantly check whether her understanding is consistent with the theories of the Grid or whether she has allowed the various Grid positions to gravitate and interpret them from her own subjective point of view.

The latter is very unfortunate, and this kind of Grid salad results in a person remaining unclear as to what constitutes sound 9,9 management, administration, and supervision.

SUMMARY

Each of these compound theories recognizes the dilemma of getting production with and through people. Each tries in some way to handle it. However, compound theories distort the basic possibility of integrating people into production, with all of the benefits available from doing so. Their underlying limitations are that they do not seek to change the status quo, and therefore, by trying to adjust to it, *deal* with symptoms rather than *correct* underlying causes. The real solution lies in learning to apply principles of human behavior to involve people in work and to integrate their individual goals and the goals of the organization with one another in a 9,9-oriented way.

Chapter 9

DIAGNOSING YOUR DOMINANT AND BACKUP GRID STYLES

The utility of the Grid is in the framework it provides a nursing administrator to sharpen her Grid-related perceptions of herself as an administrator. With these self-perceptions she is in a position to make judgments about the possible contribution that behavioral adjustments could make toward improving her effectiveness.

The chapters up to now have provided a basis for seeing Grid styles. This chapter provides two diagnostic approaches useful for evaluating your own dominant and backup Grid styles. One is the Grid mirror you filled out in Chapter 2. The second is a methodology of self-report where you apply the Grid framework to show how you see yourself.

PART 1: GRID STYLE SELF-ASSESSMENT

First, in Chapter 2 you ranked all of the sentences grouped under each of the six elements. These elements are *decisions, convictions, conflict, temper, humor,* and *energetic enthusiasm.*

You may want to rerank the elements from most to least typical as descriptions of your behavior. Again, 5 is most typical, 4 is the next most typical, and so on to 1, which is least typical. When you finish ranking the elements there should be only one of each number, from 5 to 1, and there can be no ties.

Now transfer to Figure 2 your rankings from the Grid elements listed in Chapter 2. Total each column. The column with the largest number represents your dominant Grid style, the next largest your backup Grid style, and so on. How do you see yourself? Are you oriented in the 9,9 direction? Or, is the 9,1; 1,9; 1,1; or 5,5 orientation most characteristic of you? If your answer is 9,9, is that the real you?

A word of caution. Self-deception may have occurred when you made your rankings because everyone finds it difficult to make a distinction between what "sounds good" as a self-description and what is an accurate self-description. The deception is caused by the tendency of people to confuse the way they

Element	Grid style				
	1,1	1,9	5,5	9,1	9,9
1 Decisions	A1____	B1____	C1____	D1____	E1____
2 Convictions	A2____	B2____	C2____	D2____	E2____
3 Conflict	A3____	B3____	C3____	D3____	E3____
4 Temper	A4____	B4____	C4____	D4____	E4____
5 Humor	A5____	B5____	C5____	D5____	E5____
6 Energetic enthusiasm	A6____	B6____	C6____	D6____	E6____
Total	____	____	____	____	____

Fig. 2. Summary of personal rankings.

want to be with the way they *are*. The importance of objectivity in self-description would be hard to overestimate, and the fact that self-deception is widespread cannot be denied.

A nursing administrator may be unable to view her behavior objectively and accurately. Instead, she fools herself, saying her approach is a 9,9 orientation when it really is 9,1, or she confuses 5,5 organization attitudes with 9,9-oriented team achievement. She rationalizes that a 1,9 orientation of sweetness and light really gets staff members involved. A nursing administrator may even delude herself into believing that a 1,1 orientation is the right way to settle back and emotionally quit when she looks at all the problems with which she has to contend.

These rationalizations and self-explanations are caused by many background factors. Among them is the fact that many people simply have not had the opportunity to reflect and to develop a thoughtful view as to what constitutes sound behavior. As a result, whatever they have learned from parents, teachers, or friends is accepted more or less at face value and relied upon without critical evaluation. The fact that some of what has been learned may contradict other aspects of what has been learned is not readily apparent to the person, and therefore she can embrace contradictory notions at different times and without realizing it.[8]

An indication of self-deception is that fifty percent of respondents change their self-description when they compare the way they see themselves after having studied the Grid in a deeper way. The first step in accurate self-assessment is to strip away self-deception in order to understand the underlying assumptions on which one's approach to life is based. Some self-deception is probably unavoidable, although it can be reduced by selecting answers based on your actual performance.

A questionnaire is the starting point of your diagnosis. Interviewing yourself, you now probe for the true degree of self-understanding. Finally, you develop your assessment as to how severe, strong, or extreme is the particular dominant theory (or double dominant theories) on which your behavior is based.

The best way to conduct this interview is to ask yourself, for example, "Why did I pick the D statement as most typical of me in my daily life?" Your answer might be, "Because that seems to be the best description of how I conduct myself." You might ask yourself, "Why was the D statement better than the C statement as a description of myself? What's wrong with the C statement as my first choice?" (This is a particularly good point to ask yourself if the "D" paragraph is ranked 5 and the "C" paragraph is ranked 4.) You might answer by saying, "Well, the C statement is also characteristic of me, but it is not as typical. I do behave that way sometimes, but I think my behavior is more like the D statement most of the time." Then you ask yourself, "Can I give myself an example of D behavior?" When you come up with an example, you will want to reconstruct this incident and probe into it to ensure that it is valid and, if it is not, then to select another statement which might better describe the actual behavior.

You will find that "testing the limits" of your self-perceptions is also very useful in the following way. Whatever statement is ranked 1 is the most rejected one; that is, the statement that is most unlike how you see yourself. It is important to learn why you think that statement to be an inadequate or poor description and much can be learned by asking yourself why you reject it. Say, for example, that the most rejected statement is "B" (1,9). Then it is important to know why this orientation is rejected as being very unlike you. You might ask yourself, "Why did I reject the B statement?" The answer might be, "That sounds like sweetness and light, and if there is anything I don't do, it's to strive to be warm and loving. I hate saccharin people, who don't really make the maximum effort to get results." Should you go on and tell yourself that what is killing the world is weak people, that you deplore them to an extreme degree, the possibility is that you are telling yourself something very important about your selection of the "D," or 9,1, statement as most self-characteristic. People who do not strive to control, master, and dominate are threatening, and this may be because they are not out to win at all costs, as you may be.

The most important element from the standpoint of understanding yourself is concerned with *conflict*. This element is the centerpiece of human adjustment. The reason is that conflict is at the core of human affairs. How you deal with conflict tells much about how you relate to the world. It is therefore of significance that the conflict element be thoroughly examined during your self-assessment and that you are satisfied that you have a clear understanding of why the element is ranked as it is, with any changes in ranking reached as a result of your self-interview.

To provide an example of how the interview may be conducted, it might be most useful to concentrate upon the conflict element. One way of probing this area might be as follows.

> **Q:** "When a staff member goes against what you have asked her to do, how do you handle it? Describe what you would do."
> **A:** "I give her a piece of my mind in no uncertain terms . . . "
> **Q:** "Do you swear?"
> **A:** "Sometimes, when I lose my temper. You can see that in the way I ranked the sentences in that area."
> **Q:** "After it is all over, does this roll off like water from a duck's back, or do you continue to think about it?"
> **A:** "I think about it, brood on it, and worry about it."
> **Q:** "How does it affect your sleep?"
> **A:** "Many times I toss and turn, unable to get it out of my mind, and this also increases my anger toward her."
> **Q:** "What about conflict with your spouse (or children)?"

This exploration then permits you to test for the consistency of the pattern between your manner of resolving conflict with a staff member in comparison with your manner of dealing with conflict with your spouse or children.

If the same pattern is repeated, this tells a significant amount about the generality of your approach whenever someone goes against you. On the other hand, it may be found that another element is selected in answering questions about "How do you solve conflict problems with your spouse?" in comparison with ". . . your staff member?"

There are many subtle aspects of diagnosis, but these cannot be dealt with further at this time. Suggestions for the important things for the self-diagnostician to be on the lookout for are available elsewhere, as are open seminars useful for deepening your skills in this area.[9]

PART 2: GRID STYLE CLUE SHEET

Next we turn to your self-observations. This section contains a series of sentences that you can use to characterize the Grid style you observed in yourself as you think about details of everyday working with and through other people.

Clue sheet instructions

Following are clues to help you in making an analysis of your Grid style as you go about your everyday work. Evaluate each item for the extent to which it describes you. The maximum number of points you can assign any statement is 9, and the maximum total for any Grid theory is 90. The minimum you can assign any statement is 1, and the minimum total to any Grid theory is 10.

A CLUE SHEET

Score

_____ Appear more or less indifferent to the whole of nursing administration.

_____ Seem quite passive and follow more than lead conversations.

_____ Do not show much interest in other individuals.

_____ Volunteer little or no information. When I am asked a question, I give something of an answer and then close up again.

_____ Try to appear interested in most activities, but it is an act.

_____ Don't seem to have feelings, one way or the other.

_____ Seem something like a bore, and my job is something of a chore.

_____ Don't find my work experiences to be very much fun.

_____ Accept just about any answer anyone gives me as okay.

_____ Seem to get discouraged easily and to almost prefer to leave something undone rather than to continue the effort.

_____ Total

B CLUE SHEET

Score

_____ Convey a sweet and warm attitude, smiling frequently, and agreeing wherever possible.

_____ Act as though I feel the need to be loved.

_____ Take pleasure in telling everything I am asked.

_____ Am paid compliments, and getting them makes me feel more secure.

_____ Say things I think others want to hear.

_____ Seem to dread mentioning anything that might be interpreted as negative.

_____ Fear being rejected.

_____ Want to please.

_____ Act with deference.

_____ Am almost too polite.

_____ Total

C CLUE SHEET

Score

_____ Seem to want to impress others regarding my status, reputation, and prestige.

_____ Seem quite tentative rather than giving flat answers.

_____ Don't push but keep testing as to the acceptability of my tempo.

_____ Seem to worry about giving a "wrong" answer and so appear somewhat cautious.

_____ See external appearances as important, based on dress and manners.

_____ Seem to be an active but shallow thinker.

_____ Explain myself in stereotypical terms.

_____ Seem to feel I can make an impression by being entertaining.

_____ Keep my answers open-ended so I can "shift" without losing face.

_____ Seem to give "answers" that are prosaic.

_____ Total

D CLUE SHEET

Score

_____ Come on too strong and overwhelm subordinates.

_____ Control the conversation by monopolizing, and when not monopolizing, correcting points with which others might have been in disagreement, no matter how trivial.

_____ Seem to resent questions.

_____ Seem free to fire questions at staff members at any time, even though this may interrupt the flow of conversation.

_____ Seem to admire aggressive behavior.

_____ Almost push conversations into a win-lose battle.

_____ Don't seem to be too concerned about feelings.

_____ Tend to raise objections to whatever is being said.

_____ Try to wear others down.

_____ Control the conversation, and expect others to fit in.

_____ Total

E CLUE SHEET

Score

_____ Am respected by my subordinates.

_____ Enjoy everyday give-and-take with staff members.

_____ Get right down to brass tacks at the beginning of the work day and stay on track.

_____ Give enough personal detail about myself or my thinking to help get the "what the real problem is" question into perspective.

_____ Listen keenly. Facts and logic seem to register with me.

_____ Request clarification whenever a statement appears vague or unclear.

_____ Pose comments and questions, but do not distract when relevant points are already being made.

_____ Realize that completing projects often is a two-way result of cooperation.

_____ Am open and friendly. There is no need to withhold or become defensive.

_____ Have an authentic quality.

_____ Total

The Grid style clue sheets are organized in the same sequence of Grid styles as are the statements to the elements. Thus the order of the statements within each element and the order of Grid styles in the clue sheet is as follows: 1,1 (A) followed by 1,9 (B), 5,5 (C), 9,1 (D), and 9,9 (E).

Another step that can now be taken involves comparing the answers in terms of your dominant and backup Grid styles from the Grid element study with the behavioral description that you have just completed. Since there are ten statements in each Grid clue section, the maximum that you can score on any Grid style is 90 and the minimum is 10. Does the Grid style that earned the maximum score for you in Part 1 square with the Grid style that earned the maximum in Part 2? They should. If they do not, then you need to deal with why they do not parallel one another. It may be that self-deception was stronger in completing the Grid elements than it was in describing how you see your own behavior with staff members. You may now wish to revise the sentence rankings that you did in Part 1.

In any event, the answers to the dominant Grid style in Part 1 should be parallel by the same style being dominant in Part 2. This also applies for backups. The theory that you said was your backup theory in Part 1 should also be found to have the second highest score in the self-description work that you have just completed in Part 2.

Having completed your self-assessment, you are in a position to take a further step to corroborate your conclusions. After you have developed hypotheses as to (1) your dominant orientation, (2) your backup orientation, and (3) the intensity or extremeness of these orientations, another step is to evaluate your findings by asking loved ones or intimate acquaintances to picture you. This can also be done through having the intimate acquaintances complete the paragraph and element study, and it may be done in terms of asking the intimate acquaintance to use the Grid Style Clue Sheet as the basis for picturing your adjustment. The option is to simply ask questions, the answers to which verify or invalidate the hypotheses you have already formulated.

CAN YOU CHANGE?

Thirty years ago people often said, "Life begins at forty." But in the era of the eighties you are over the hill at thirty, according to the "now" generation. What is meant is that most people have become complacent, stuck in their ruts, and, as a consequence, unable to change significantly after reaching thirty. Whether life begins at forty or stops at thirty has nothing to do with bones, muscles, nerves, and blood. It has everything to do with a person's point of view. An individual can get crusty and dead from the neck up at twenty or can be lively, creative, enthusiastic, and growing professionally at sixty.

Comparison learning

Learning is essential for change, so it is important to know more about conditions that are favorable for bringing about personal improvement.

Conditions are favorable for learning whenever a person can make comparisons between two or more things. Then similarities and differences can be examined, the reasons for them analyzed, and a determination made of which of the two is better in terms of relative merit. When you see similarities and differences, understand the reasons beneath the surface, and can evaluate them on a "degrees of good and bad" basis, you are then in a position to plot a course of action for how to get from where you are to where you want to be.

Now take this concept of how learning occurs and apply it to changing your Grid style, if that is what you want to do, or to strengthening the one you have, if that is the conclusion you have reached. First of all, the Grid itself provides the basis for a series of comparisons. In many different ways, as you have read this book, you have been comparing a 9,9 orientation with the other styles of behavior. You can see the similarities between the 9,1 and 9,9 orientations. One is that both have a high concern for getting results. A 9,1 orientation disregards the patient as a unique and distinctive individual, while a 9,9 approach appreciates the individual as the person for whom the nursing administrator should have the utmost respect. This is the key difference.

Also similar are 1,9 and 1,1 orientations. Neither of them has much concern for getting results, but a nursing administrator with a 1,9 attitude enjoys people, whereas the 1,1-oriented nursing administrator is indifferent to them. Thus there are similarities and differences here, too. A 5,5-oriented nursing administrator, in comparison with all others, shares some basic similarities but some very important differences. In some respects, this person approaches a 9,9 orientation, but the major difference is that this style is shallow and mechanical rather than deep and committed. This is the fundamental basis for comparison.

Comparison of Grid positions

A first step in strengthening yourself is to possess a clear understanding with regard to Grid concepts. Here is how you can test yourself. Take some particular supervisory situation that you now have, and write down what the 9,1 attitude toward that situation would be. Then move on and describe the 1,9 attitude. What would be the 1,1 reaction? How would a 5,5-oriented nursing administrator think about the situation? Finally, picture the 9,9 approach to dealing with it.

Taking your own statements, you might then want to switch back to parts of this book that are related to the same or similar situations and test your statements against the text. You might want to change some and refine others. You will find that writing statements in this way will aid you in diagnosing various ways of seeing a supervisory situation and therefore in dealing with it. If you will do this from time to time, you will find that it continues strengthening your understanding of the Grid. It will help you in self-diagnosis, because you will be able to see alternative ways of dealing with the situation that might differ from your present approach.

Comparing your attitudes with the Grid

You can compare and analyze similarities and differences among these five major orientations, but, of course, there is something far more important if you want to change or strengthen yourself. This involves comparing your own attitudes with those of the Grid and seeing which Grid orientation corresponds most closely with your own. This will tell you where you are. You did this to some extent earlier on the elements and clue sheets. A second step is to come to your own conclusions as to why you are there and then decide whether this is where you want to be. In making your decision, it is helpful to analyze which Grid styles are not at all like you. This is important because it will tell you something about your aversions. Once you understand what it is you dislike, you very well may want to ask yourself if you act poorly with staff members who represent in their Grid styles the Grid style you reject in yourself. This aids you to see why some persons bother you, and you can discover new ways for working more effectively with those who represent aspects of behavior you dislike. The chances are that, once you understand your own feelings and actions, you will find it possible to be more constructive and positive in working with people.

Choosing what is ideal

There is still another way you can use the Grid as the basis for self-development. It involves identifying the Grid style that fits you best. This is the one that you think would be ideal as the most effective way of supervising. Go even further—identify the soundest backup you can adopt and the type of situation that would impel you to use it. Knowing the Grid description that currently fits you best—as you have been operating—and knowing the Grid style that would be best in terms of effectiveness provide the basis for you to set development objectives for yourself. In making this comparison between the actual you and the ideal you, you will be able to see what you do that is sound and what you do that is not. It also increases your awareness of what you do not do that you would need to do if you were to act in a truly sound way.

Assume that you selected the 9,9 orientation as the ideal, for this is the most likely possibility. No matter how sound any particular Grid style you chose might seem to be, it is realistic only insofar as it is workable. Even though 9,9 is a practical, problem-solving approach that you are probably capable of adopting and to which most persons can respond favorably, there are situations in which a 9,9 orientation—or any style you adopt as the soundest—may be unworkable. Your skill in supervising under this approach may be insufficient. In a particular situation, the behavior of your staff member may be such as to obstruct completely your chosen approach. In situations such as these, you have no choice but to move into a backup strategy until you see an opportunity to return to the dominant style that you have found to be the soundest under most conditions.

The real test in self-development is learning to increase the versatility with which 9,9 solutions can be implemented, so that it seldom is necessary to adopt backup assumptions. You may also find ways to initiate and take part in constructive discussion and improvement of your hospital and its policies and procedures.

Ask your spouse

If you are married you can also do this kind of data gathering about yourself by giving this book to your wife or husband. Your spouse undoubtedly knows you as well and perhaps better than anyone else, in terms of what turns you on and what turns you off, what you will accept and what you cannot take. Ask your mate to read the book and then to return to Chapter 2, picking out elements that are most typical of you. You can gain a great deal of good understanding of yourself through your spouse's eyes. Incidentally, you may find that this has some very good effects on your marriage. Many people have found the Grid a useful way of analyzing how husband and wife exert influence on one another and also how both act with regard to children.

Grid seminars for nursing administrators

Another way to gain insight into your Grid styles as a nursing administrator is through a seminar at which nursing administrators are helped to learn their Grid styles in a clear and objective way, and can practice the skills of change necessary for shifting from one Grid style to a 9,9 orientation.

The Nursing Grid Seminar, for example, designed specifically for this purpose, consists of ten modules, each taking three hours to complete. The minimum number of participants recommended in any given module is four, but two or three teams of four persons each, working simultaneously, have been found to be the most functional. This special training emphasizes the important key points of contact between nursing administrators and staff members in pursuit of heightened production. These include communication, handling mistakes, giving directions, dealing with complaints, reacting to hostile feelings, and performance evaluation.[10]

SUMMARY

This chapter has been introduced in order to aid you to make a first approximation in identifying your dominant and backup Grid style.

Two approaches to self-assessment were introduced.

One of these involved you in ranking Grid elements and evaluating these in such a way as to reveal your dominant and backup Grid style.

The second way asked you to describe how you see yourself in your everyday activities of administration.

These two different approaches should agree. You should get the same answer from both, but if you do not, it may be helpful to return to Chapter 8, Combinations of Grid Theories, to see if you can identify reasons for these discrepancies.

A third way of developing insight into your own dominant and backup Grid styles was suggested, which involves asking that the form used in Part 1 and the form used in Part 2 be completed by an intimate acquaintance to picture how that person sees you as an administrator. Here, too, the results should be consistent with those that you have already produced to picture yourself. If they are not, you then need to explore with your intimate acquaintance why he or she filled in the two parts as was done. This may help in reducing self-deception.

The fourth, and in many ways the best, way to learn about one's Grid style as an administrator is to attend a seminar specifically designed to further such understanding in the development of skills in implementing a more 9,9 orientation.

Chapter 10

THE ADMINISTRATIVE NURSE
IN THE HEALTH DELIVERY SYSTEM

HISTORICAL PERSPECTIVE

Historically the nurse has been seen by doctors and the public as a doer, carrying out a special set of techniques, hence a technical nurse. This is now beginning to change.[11] Recently posters appeared showing pictures of Florence Nightingale, Clara Barton, and other past nurse leaders with a statement under the pictures saying, in effect, "You now know more than Florence Nightingale and Clara Barton did in their day." The knowledge explosion—the new medical research sciences, educational preparation, the contributions made by physics, new surgical methods, etc.—means that preparation of the nurse of today is entirely different from say even five years ago. She is needed more than ever, and the difference is more than just giving a bed bath or taking blood pressure. There are many additional skills the nurse of today is capable of helping the medical staff implement.

What about the patient as a human being who needs compassion and touch? The nurse who knows how to help the patient strengthen his or her resolve toward health is vital to meet the demands of the nursing profession in the next decade.

Unfortunately some directors of nursing, head nurses, and charge nurses are trying to administer patient care as was done in the past. All this newness is very bewildering to them. They want to cope with all the changes but cannot understand modern education or the modern nurse. Some of these persons still have influence in the hospitals, yet hospitals are a twentieth century phenomena. As society has changed to absorb new knowledge, hospitals have found that they too must change.

EVOLUTIONARY TRENDS

Take a look at history. In the early days, the organization consisted of a director of nurses or the superintendent who had the help of some supervisors and head nurses.[12] Student nurses did all the work. Besides being there to learn, they took care of patients, the stove, the floors, etc. A head nurse was simply chosen from the students on graduation and thrown into the situation to make it all come together.

Most graduate nurses became private duty nurses or worked in the operating room. As nursing schools were organized, graduate nurses became members of the faculty to teach the next generation how to give patient care and how to organize the nursing function. Yet the supervisor or the head nurse never really had the opportunity to prepare for their positions. It was not unusual, upon being appointed as a head nurse, to be told by a supervisor "A good head nurse runs her unit from the desk." The more autocratic the leader, the better it was felt the hospital was being run.

Changes began to take place in the preparation of nurses after World War II. Student nurses no longer were used as "free labor." The GI Bill encouraged many veteran nurses to take courses and to obtain baccalaureate degrees. Many college schools of nursing offered courses in nursing management as a first recognition that nursing leaders needed preparation in administration. As changes began to take place in industry, so changes began to take place in hospitals: for example, the organization chart, job descriptions, wage scales, personnel policies, and no more exploitation of workers.[13]

Unfortunately, the National League of Nursing concluded in this era that university programs should deemphasize preparation of administrators and emphasize the preparation of clinical specialists. With the NLN as the accrediting body, the majority of university schools of nursing complied. We are now realizing the error of this decision because the majority of nursing administrators, regardless of hospital size, are not prepared for their positions.

Many universities are now offering a functional major in nursing service as administration. This trend will continue, and it will become easier for staff and head nurses to become administrative professionals. Then, too, the better prepared top administration is, the easier it is for the entire staff to function in a sound manner. Changes can be introduced as needed, and the staff nurse can think about them as well as help implement them.

Another group of people need to be mentioned. These are the patients, the consumers of health care. Years ago, patients were brought into the hospital but were not allowed to ask questions. They were told exactly what to do, and if they did not follow orders, they could switch doctors or leave. All this is now changing. Patients are more well read. They understand diseases. They know what is going on in their bodies. They dare to ask questions. They are no longer bewildered by the doctor. They will, if necessary, seek another doctor's advice if this is thought to be needed. When it comes to the nurse-patient relationship, patients expect nurses to respond to, and to answer, their questions.

What does all of this add up to when it comes to nursing administration? It is no longer feasible for a director of nursing, a head nurse, or a charge nurse simply to tell others what to do and expect them to do it. Professional people do not act that way, and the patient care staff nurse is a true professional. A whole new way of supervision is now necessary. It means that the nursing administrator has the skills necessary for gaining the involvement, participation, and commitment of those for whom she is responsible. It means supervising a hospital in such a way that patient care is provided according to the highest standards and, in doing so, earning the patients' respect for her competence, understanding, support, and genuine helpfulness.

BARRIERS TO CHANGE

But change is not always possible. The reason is that factors exist outside and beyond the administrative nurse's control that impose requirements on her, and these are requirements that she cannot ignore. Therefore, the situation in which she is embedded may be a deterrent to change. We need to study and understand this and see what can be done about it.

No head nurse (director of nurses, etc.) is an island unto herself. This paraphrase of a well-known quotation emphasizes the point that no nurse administrator works in a vacuum. Many variables surround and control the director of nursing and the head nurse. These include hospital administrators, doctors, other department heads, and many other hospital personnel. These all may have an influence on the Grid style that she may be forced to rely on by circumstances. Examples of this will be found in the text that follows.

The hospital administrator

A director of nurses may be told by hospital administration, "This new policy is already in effect. Inform your staff. There will be no questions. Do it!" A 9,1-oriented director of nurses relates this dictum verbatim to her staff. The 1,9-oriented nurse apologizes and may blame "them" (administration), but still she has no option but to "do it." A 1,1-oriented nurse hopes it will all blow over, but she has no option but to "do it." A 5,5-oriented nurse takes no sides if she can help it, but hopes others will not resist her message to "do it." The 9,9-oriented nurse relates the dictum to her staff but also says, "I'm sorry, but that's the new policy, and we're going to have to live with it. You can react to it, but I can't do anything about it." This works against her philosophy of leading but it is only acknowledging a fact of her life.

The doctor

The doctor is a different breed unto himself. In spite of the fact that a doctor typically has no authority as far as an organizational chart is concerned, he or she is very influential and can be demanding, making nursing personnel miserable.

Some doctors are excellent surgeons. No matter the skill in surgery, sometimes they have demanding personalities. These medical experts usually are tolerated, and even admired, because of their great technical skill. Such doctors can make unusual and varied demands on the nursing staff and gain cooperation because of the nurse's admiration for competence.

Other doctors, themselves less skilled, may make unusual and varied demands and not get cooperation. Some head nurses may challenge them, but the doctor in turn can say, "Do as I say." The director of nurses or the head nurse may not always be backed by administration when doctors make unreasonable demands. In many hospitals, the doctor can take all their patients to another hospital if they feel put upon by the nurses. If this is the only hospital in the town or city, the nursing administrator may have to compromise. She is stuck, which may cause her to become a 1,1.

There are times when nurses go to doctors with their complaints against the "system" rather than go through the proper channels if they think they cannot get what they think they need. It is not unusual for doctors to call the director of nursing and relay to her some of these complaints. In an insidious way this only adds to their "unofficial" power. If a doctor complains to a weak director of nurses, she always tends to take the doctor's side against the head nurse.

All these influences can "cause" a nursing administrator to embrace a Grid style that gets results, at least short term, no matter how she may deplore such demands.

Director of nurses

Most head nurses do not make totally independent decisions. They usually have to get an okay from the director of nurses or the doctor.

Conflict often arises when the head nurse is better prepared technically than the director of nurses herself. That can happen when the head nurse is a baccalaureate graduate versus a diploma held by the director of nurses or the supervisor. Not having the same educational background, a director of nurses may reflect the wishes of those above her, unwilling to support a head nurse's efforts, especially a 9,9-oriented one. The director may be suspicious of participation and involvement of the staff, which in turn blocks the head nurse's efforts to administer in a sounder way.

Other departments

Other departments complain, and the nursing administrator often gets the blame. No one really inquires as to "why" the patient is not prepared right, or whether things do not go well with dietary, or whether patients are not prepared to eat. The head nurse gets the blame almost regardless of extenuating circumstances.

For example, it is not unusual for labs to discard specimens, saying that the unit did not send one. The head nurse is "blamed." If the new head nurse or staff nurse wants to do some research or test new ideas, they have to be cleared with a great many people, including doctors, who may refuse because they think the nurse will become too powerful. Or the director of nurses refuses because she may not want to see anything changed. So we have nurses right in the middle—wanting to take initiative but being blocked from doing so—and this has a controlling effect on the nursing administrator's Grid style.

What has been pointed out brings us to quite a different issue of effectiveness. The issue is that the hospital system itself may have traditions, precedents, and past practices, built in frictions between departments or between levels, and tensions between the administration and the trustees. All of these are potential deterrents to the administrative nurse's effectiveness. The nursing department is, of course, no exception. It is a component in the larger system; therefore, the department as a whole and its individual administrators are influenced by the culture of the hospital itself, and in turn its own traditions, precedents, and past practices influence exercise of initiative and ways of responding to initiatives from other departments.

CHANGING THE CULTURE OF A HOSPITAL

More and more organization leaders are coming to realize that the entire hospital system is subject to self-study and to change by those who manage and work within it. This has led to the concept of organization development for the hospital.

The Grid approach to hospital organization development is based on the New Managerial Grid.[14] The Managerial Grid is a study of many of the issues that are involved in exercising power and authority throughout an entire institutional system such as a hospital. Grid Organization Development is built on and develops through a series of six phases. Each is briefly described in the following pages.

Grid learning: Phase 1

In the initial phase of organization development everyone in management gets involved in learning the Grid and using it to evaluate their own personal style of managing. This learning and self-study is through attending a seminar.

Maximum impact is possible when all employees participate. Included are persons who manage others, though some organizations extend participation in organization development to include technical, wage, and salaried personnel. The decision on extending Grid learning to other than managerial levels can be made at a later time.

These seminars are conducted on both an external and an internal basis.

They involve hard work. The program consists of thirty or more hours of guided study before the seminar week itself.

The sessions include investigation by participants of their own managerial approach and alternate ways of managing, which they are able to experiment with, test out, and apply. Participants experience and study team action, measuring and evaluating team effectiveness in solving problems. A high point of seminar learning is when participants receive a critique of their style of managerial performance from other team members. Another is when managers critique the dominant style of their organization's culture, that is, traditions, precedents, and past practices. A third is when participants consider steps for increasing the effectiveness of the whole organization.

Team building: Phase 2

Phase 2, Team Building, begins when all members of any hospital team have completed Phase 1, Grid learning, and decide to apply concepts for evaluating and changing their own team's culture. To do this, each manager sits with his or her subordinates as a team. They study their barriers to effectiveness and plan ways to overcome them. It starts with the key executive and those who report to him or her, and then moves down through the organization.

An analysis of team culture and operating practices precedes the setting of goals for improvement of the team, along with a time schedule for achieving these goals. Members learn how to become more productive through synergizing their individual contributions. Sound and enduring standards of excellence are established as benchmarks for the team's use in continually strengthening its problem-solving culture. Tied into the goal setting for the team is personal goal setting by individual members. A demonstration project is selected to enable the team to immediately apply its new openness and problem-solving skills and standards to solve a significant barrier to effectiveness with which it is faced in everyday work.

Grid Team Building is a five-day activity. It is conducted on the job during working hours. If job considerations require it, the activities can be segmented into parts and conducted over a longer period.

Development of improved interdepartmental relationships: Phase 3

The next step is to achieve better problem solving between groups through a closer integration of units that have working interrelationships. The need for Phase 3 development comes about because, when each department or unit has a singular responsibility, members of departments tend to think more about their components and less about the other departments or the hospital as an organic whole. Because the nursing service is so central, so large, and so continuous twenty-four hours a day, it is in a position that often results in its being in conflict with hospital services; for example, dietary, housekeeping, maintenance, lab, x-ray, administration, bookkeeping, and accounting. These conflicts are most likely to erupt during the night and over the weekend when other personnel are not on duty. People can see most clearly what they experience, their most immediate interests. From inside the department, this is viewed as selflessly serving the hospital agency. They may unintentionally act and react more in the interests of their departmentalized units rather than in the interests of the entire hospital. Such preoccupation may mean that less of their attention is paid to cooperation with other departments. Then, when one department must cooperate with another, managers in the second tend to see those in the first motivated by selfish considerations.

Phase 3 is participated in only by those departments in which actual barriers to effective cooperation exist. It is not a "universal" phase that all members automatically engage in. Intergroup development usually is undertaken after Phase 2 Grid team building has been completed.

Designing an ideal strategic organization model: Phase 4

When Phases 1 through 3 have been completed, many outmoded traditions, precedents, and past practices have already been replaced by standards of excellence for judging individual performance and effective teamwork and for confronting and resolving cleavages between groups. This is important to organization excellence, but none of it is sufficient for reaching the degree of excellence potentially available. The systematic development of strategic, operational logic employed throughout an organization for strengthening productivity is an additional step toward outstanding hospital administration.

The key to exploiting potentials for excellence is in the organization having a model of what it wishes to become in comparison with what it currently is or historically has been.

The top team of an organization is ideally situated for carrying out such a fundamental study for examining and rejecting whatever in its current practices is outmoded and unprofitable and formulating a replacement model. The model is based on the organization's being engaged in activity in the future that is geared to the needs of society for sound health delivery, and the needs of employees for satisfaction with work based upon involvement, participation, and commitment.

Designing an ideal strategic organization model is a planning technique that enables the top team to apply rigorous, operational logic in blueprinting what the organization is expected to become during its next stage of development.

Implementing development: Phase 5

The Phase 5 activity moves an organization out of its traditional ways of operating and into alignment with the ideal strategic model. Phase 5 is designed so that it is unnecessary to tear down the whole organization and start from scratch to build a new one to meet the requirements of the model. What is done is more like remodeling a building according to a blueprint of what it is to become. Then architects and engineers study the existing structure to identify what is strong, sound, and consistent with the blueprint and can be retained, what is antiquated and inappropriate to the blueprint and must be replaced, and what is usable but needs modification or strengthening in order to bring it into line. Once these decisions have been reached, then carpenters, plumbers, and others know what must be done concretely to shift from the old to the new. The professionals who do this are the ones who operate the hospital, including the director of nurses and the head nurse.

Consolidation: Phase 6

Phase 6 is a period that is used to stabilize and to consolidate progress achieved during Phases 1 through 5 before recycling into another period of change and development.

Three features of hospital management suggest the importance of a consolidating phase in organization development. Managing change is the opposite of managing the tried and true. People tend to repeat the tried and true, but people may lose enthusiasm and confidence in attempting something that is novel and that they are less familiar with. Reduced effort in making the novel work as it is intended may cause it to fail. Phase 6 activities help to identify these drag factors that tend to pull an organization in a backward direction.

A second reason for spending a period of time in order to consolidate progress is that, by continuing the study of what is new, additional improvement opportunities may be identified that can add to the organizational thrust. A third reason is that significant alterations in the outer environment may occur to cause changes specified in the model and implemented in Phase 5 to be more or less favorable than had been anticipated. In either case the monitoring activities of Phase 6 provide a basis for specifying the needs for additional change.

Phase 6 strategies and instruments enable an organization to assess its strengths and to consolidate its gains. This is done by organization members identifying drag factors that may have cropped up and that need to be eliminated to counter their adverse effects. The same is true for thrust factors. These may need to be stressed in order to gain the full potential of organization development. The significant aspect of Phase 6 is that the consolidation phase is made explicit rather than those in charge assuming that once change has been set in motion, it will persist of its own momentum. Often the influences that are adverse to effective patient care impact on the nursing department and stem from influences that are external to it and above it. Thus, bringing better nursing to its patient population is contingent upon the leadership and the other departments of the hospital learning to change the culture of this entire delivery system.

NURSING IN THE FUTURE

Many influences point toward the 9,9 direction of nursing excellence. Nursing education constantly on the march provides new insight and skills, introduces new possibilities, and excites new appetites for something better than what now exists. Cultural concepts of excellence leave people uneasy with conditions that fail to match what they know is attainable. Standards from advanced education place high value on doing things in the best way.

Another trend is the steady improvement of merit-based compensation systems that result in their rewarding 9,9 contribution and commitment that lead to relations that are open, communicative, and problem solving rather than closed, suspicious, and problem generating. The university has provided a mechanism whereby nursing can shift away from the medical model of teaching nurses how to care for and view patients. They are beginning to use all other kinds of methods: the adaptation process, the holistic point of view, and therapeutic touch. These are methods that nursing has used to teach students a better understanding of patients. If we look back at the previous quote, "Nurses now know more than . . . " nurses now know a lot more than nurses knew ten, even five years ago.

The search goes on unceasingly for better ways to supervise. As important as any factor in establishing 9,9 as a dynamic trend is the emergence of applied behavioral science education within industry through organization development. These methods, coupled with a growing body of behavioral science concepts, have been readily accepted by hospitals, and it is not unusual to find many hospitals bringing in management consultants and sending personnel to human relations seminars so that they will better understand sound ways of working with one another.[15]

In addition to a wider application of all the principles we mentioned previously, nursing is seeing its members receive higher compensation, merit rewards, and greater status. Education of nurses has now leveled off at baccalaureate, masters, and doctorate levels. Each of these levels is making contributions to practice and to implementing new modalities of service to individuals, groups, organizations, and larger social systems.

Those who have studied and experimented with a 9,9 orientation as an organization style in hospitals and medical centers recognize that it is attainable. Those who come by it naturally know what they want. They want the self-respect that comes from respect for others at work. They want meaningful relationships that only mutual respect built around common purposes can sustain. Better productivity, increased creativity, and greater satisfaction with work are the inevitable results.

Nursing personnel are very much concerned about the care that their patients receive, and many of them feel that a 9,9 approach may be the answer. The trend toward a 9,9 orientation is sound and the great challenge is to create conditions so that it can be brought into use on a wider scale.

SUMMARY

Managerial styles based on 9,1 direction with compliance, 5,5 conformity with compromise, 1,9 security and comfort, or 1,1 acquiescence, resignation, and abandonment are no more than second best. They are unacceptable in the long term. Compared with performance under a 9,9 orientation, with its condition of candid communication based on conviction, commitment, and creativity, and head nurse–subordinate relationships based on mutual respect, other approaches fall far short. The deeper trends of social evolution seem to move in directions that add meaning to mental effort and social experience. A 9,9 orientation defines a trend leading to mature relationships. Many organizations seem to be moving in this direction.

REFERENCES AND
SUGGESTED READINGS

References

1. Finer, Herman: Administration and the nursing services, New York, 1961, Macmillan, Inc.
2. The literature of behavioral science research on which the Grid is based includes about 400 references. The sources of these references are Blake, Robert R., and Mouton, Jane Srygley; The managerial Grid, Houston, 1964, Gulf Publishing Co.; and Blake, Robert R., and Mouton, Jane Srygley; The new managerial Grid, Houston, 1978, Gulf Publishing Co. (See Appendix.)
3. Blake, Robert R., and Mouton, Jane Srygley; The new Grid for supervisory effectiveness, Austin, Texas, 1978, Scientific Methods, Inc.
4. Stevens, Barbara J.: The nurse as executive, Wakefield, Mass., 1975, Contemporary Publishing, Inc.
5. Blake, Robert R., and Mouton, Jane Srygley. The new managerial Grid, Houston, 1978, Gulf Publishing Co., p. 4.

   The role of assumptions in guiding behavior is widely recognized in the behavioral sciences. Typical are Bion, W. R.: Experience in groups, New York, 1959, Basic Books, Inc., Publishers; McGregor, D.: The human side of enterprise, New York, 1960, McGraw-Hill Book Co., pp. 6-8; Steiner, C. M.: Scripts people live: transactional analysis of life scripts, New York, 1974, Bantam Books, Inc., pp. 59-111; Dreikurs, R. and Grey, L.: Logical consequences: a new approach to discipline, Des Moines, Iowa, 1968, Meredith Corp., pp. 23-27; Barber, J. D.: The presidential character: predicting performance in the White House, Englewood Cliffs, N.J., 1972, Prentice-Hall, Inc., pp. 7-9.
6. Blake, Robert R., and Mouton, Jane Srygley: The managerial Grid: an exploration of key managerial orientations, Austin, Texas, 1978, Scientific Methods, Inc. The Grid seminar prework from this publication is reproduced by permission.
7. Clark, Carolyn Chambers, and Shea, Carole A.: Management in nursing, 1979, New York, McGraw-Hill Book Co.
8. One of the observations in the development of human skills of administration and supervision is that managers, supervisors, and administrators alike need to learn to discriminate between various Grid styles and to do so in accurate terms. The importance of accuracy, of course, is that without it a person can see and call some-

thing 9,9 which, in fact, is not 9,9, or call something 1,1 which is not. It is important to be able to accurately evaluate behavior and to test the degree to which it fits each of the Grid theories in precise and objective terms. Grid distortion comes about, for example, when a 1,9-oriented administrator is likely to look at 9,9 and confuse it with a 9,1 orientation. The reason for this confusion is that the 1,9-oriented administrator, looking at the 9,9 orientation, sees the first 9, the production 9, but not what comes after it. She sees it as "tough" and it obscures her vision of the second. Thus, the high concern for production in a 9,9 orientation is misinterpreted as 9,1 because it is not seen in the context of an integrated concern for achieving high production through the involvement and commitment of those who eventually are responsible for output.

Another distortion is found among those who administer according to a 9,1 orientation. When a 9,1-oriented person looks at 9,9 she misinterprets and sees 1,9 because the 9 of concern for people is misinterpreted as soft, and it tends to obscure her perception of the first 9, the production 9.

These distortions are important because a person can use these possibilities to evaluate her own Grid style in an indirect manner by answering for herself the question, "Do I see 9,9 as 'hard,' or do I see 9,9 as 'soft'?" If the answer is "hard," then 9,9 is likely being viewed from a 1,9 orientation, and if the answer is "soft," the 9,9 orientation is likely being seen from a 9,1 perspective.

The fact is that a 9,9 orientation is neither soft nor hard; it is a sound way of integrating people into production.

9. For further information contact Scientific Methods, Inc., P. O. Box 195, Austin, Texas, 78767.
10. Ibid.
11. Barrett, Jean; Gessner, Barbara A., and Phelps, Charlene: The head nurse: her leadership role, ed. 3, New York, 1975, Appleton-Century-Crofts.
12. Arndt, Clara, and Huckabay, Loucine: Nursing administration: theory for practice with a systems approach, ed. 2, St. Louis, 1980, The C. V. Mosby Co.
13. Ibid.
14. Blake, Robert R., and Mouton, Jane Srygley: The new managerial Grid, Houston, 1978, Gulf Publishing Co.

Suggested readings

Alexander, Edythe L.: Nursing administration in the hospital health care system, ed. 2, St. Louis, 1978, The C. V. Mosby Co.

Claus, Karen E., and Bailey, June T.: Power and influence in health care: a new approach to leadership. St. Louis, 1977, The C. V. Mosby Co.

Diekelmann, Nancy L., and Broadwell, Martin M.: The new hospital supervisor, Reading, Mass., 1977, Addison-Wesley Publishing Co., Inc.

DiVincenti, Marie: Administering nursing service, ed. 2, Boston, 1977, Little, Brown & Co.

Donovan, Helen: Nursing service administration: managing the enterprise, St. Louis, 1975, The C. V. Mosby Co.

Douglas, Laura M., and Bevis, Em O.: Nursing management and leadership in action, ed. 3, St. Louis, 1979, The C. V. Mosby Co.

Ganong, Joan M., and Ganong, Warren L.: Nursing management, Germantown, Md., 1976, Aspen Systems Corp.

Kron, Thora.: The management of patient care, Philadelphia, 1976, W. B. Saunders Co.

Marriner, Ann, editor: Current perspectives in nursing management, St. Louis, 1979, The C. V. Mosby Co.

Mooth, Adelma E., and Ritvo, Miriam B.: Developing the supervisory skills of the nurse, New York, 1966, The Macmillan Co.

Rubin, Irwin M., and Fry, Ronald E.: Managing human resources in health care organizations, Reston, Va., 1978, Reston Publishing Co., Inc.

Schultz, Rockwell, and Johnson, Alton C.: Management of hospitals, New York, 1976, McGraw-Hill Book Co.

Shanks, Mary D., and Kennedy, Dorothy A.: Administration in nursing, New York, 1970, McGraw-Hill Book Co.

Stevens, Barbara J.: The nurse as executive, Wakefield, Mass., 1976, Contemporary Publishing, Inc.

Taylor, Carol D.: "The hospital patients' social dilemma," American Journal of Nursing, October, 1965.

Appendix

USE OF THE GRID TO ANALYZE BEHAVIORAL SCIENCE APPROACHES TO HUMAN RELATIONSHIPS*

The original use of the Grid to analyze interactions between significant variables of management—production and people—occurred in our efforts as consultants to understand a basic conflict in a top management group. One faction maintained, "If we don't put the pressure on for higher production we're going to sink." The other faction said, "We must ease up on the pressure and start treating people in a nicer way." Thus, a 9,1 orientation met a 1,9 orientation. This *either* production *or* people way of conceiving the problem eliminated perception of other possibililties, such as getting people involved in the importance of being more productive.

By treating these variables of production and people as independent yet interacting, we came to see many alternative ways of managing—not only 9,1 and 1,9 but also 1,1, 5,5, 9,9, paternalism, counterbalancing, two-hat, statistical 5,5, and facades.

A way of thinking about human relationships that permitted such clear comprehension and comparison of alternatives led us to believe this formulation to be of general significance for understanding other human relationships. Thus we evaluated in greater detail how others had tried to deal with the same kind of question.

We found no systematic use of two-dimensional geometric space as the foundation for conceptual analysis of assumptions about how to manage, but we were struck by the extent to which such a basis of analysis was being used, either implicitly or statistically. Theorists who used two variables *implicitly*, and without identification of the variables involved, included Horney and Fromm. Other theorists who approached the situation *statistically*, without

---

*From Blake, Robert R., and Mouton, Jane Srygley: The new managerial Grid, 1978, Houston, Gulf Publishing Co., pp. 218-231.

explicit analysis of how assumptions and therefore behavior may change as a function of the character of the interaction of these variables, included Likert and Fleishman.

The table shows the various implicit or statistical approaches for comprehending human relationships that can be fitted into a Grid framework. Several explicit efforts to modify the Grid also are included and are commented on later.

As shown in the table, regardless of their field of specialization, and with but a few exceptions, all investigators describe behavior as if relying on a two-dimensional framework. Factor analytic approaches reinforce conceptual analysis and lead to the conclusion that most meaningful variance in behavior can be accounted for by two factors.

There are exceptions, however. One is Bales, who described behavior in a three-variable geometric space, the third variable being related to an individual's acceptance or rejection of conventional authority. The added complexity did little by way of extending understanding of behavior. Another, by Schutz, added *inclusion* as a third dimension, but little use has been made of it in experimental, clinical, or applied work. Reddin and Hersey and Blanchard have added effectiveness as a third Grid dimension, but this is not a true third dimension since effectiveness is already determined by the first two and therefore is not independent of them.

There is an implicit third dimension within the Grid framework, however. It involves identification of motivation as a bipolar scale, ranging, in the 9,1 case for example, between control, mastery, and domination on the plus end to dread of failure on the minus end of the scale. While adding a third dimension of motivation introduces further clarification as to what a 9,1 or other Grid orientation is like, little in predictive utility for understanding everyday behavior is gained over that already available in a two-dimensional system. This motivation dimension is available elsewhere and is not further dealt with in this context.

A further comment of importance in understanding the Grid is the concept of *interaction*. Interaction between these variables can occur in either of two ways. The combination of any two quantities can occur in an arithmetic way. This needs to be distinguished from the fusion of two quantities in a "chemical" way. Hersey and Blanchard, for example, might see 9,9 as a combination of 9 units of tasks orientation, telling a subordinate in great detail "who, what, where, and how" added to 9 units of relationships, involving extensive compliments and appreciation expressed in response to subordinate compliance. The "chemical" view, by comparison, produces a 9,9 character of interdependence in which shared participation, involvement, and commitment produce consensus-based teamwork. In the former case, combination of variables is quantitative and arithmetical; in the latter, it is qualitative and organic, that is, the *character* of the behavior itself changes, not just relative to the amounts of the same behavior.

Because most investigations have found a two-dimensional basis sufficient and three-dimensional formulations have added little to understanding beyond that already available from the use of two, we conclude that a framework for analyzing behavior that results from two variables is a sound and sufficient basis for comprehending assumptions and practices.

Catalog of approaches to human relationships through a Grid framework

Investigator	Source	Field	9.1	1.9	1.1	5.5	9.9	Statistical 5.5	Facades	Paternalism	Other
Argyris, C.	*Management and Organizational Development: The Path from XA to YB.* New York: McGraw-Hill, 1971.	Organization Behavior	xi, xii, 6-15, 66-70, 73-74, 77-78, 85-88, 105, 107, 134, 135, 138-140			13-14, 30-34, 56-57	xi, 15-20, 21-22, 24, 42, 57-61, 67-70, 85-89		19	3, 62	
Argyris, C. & Schon, D.A.	*Theory in Practice: Increasing Professional Effectiveness.* San Francisco: Jossey-Bass, 1974.	Business Administration	66-84, 101-102, 104, 105-106, 107-108, 149-155				85-95, 101, 102, 104, 105, 106-107, 108-109				
Arkava, M.L.	*Behavior Modification: A Procedural Guide for Social Workers.* Missoula: U of Montana, 1974	Social Work	16-66					1-11		1-82	
Bach, G.R. & Wyden, P.	*The Intimate Enemy.* New York: William Morrow and Company, Inc., 1969.	Psychology	8-9, 45-46, 48-49, 71-73, 75, 83, 109-117, 129, 141-150, 256-257, 311, 312, 314	5, 48, 71-73, 84-85, 97, 102-108, 311, 314, 321-322	31-32, 312	5, 53-54, 135-136	36, 43, 53, 91, 119-123, 137, 161-165, 257-258, 343-348		7, 10, 13, 19, 36, 103, 120, 159, 196-197, 222-223, 253-254	113	Sick 9.1 112-113, 151, 158, 160, 260 Distorted 1.9:75, 112, 154, 158, 160, 260, 331 Change 173-174
Bales, R.F.	*Personality and Interpersonal Behavior.* New York: Holt, Rinehart & Winston, 1970.	Sociology	193-199, 213-219, 220-229, 230-237.	200-207, 252-257, 313-319, 320-326, 369-376	289-296, 332-339, 340-346, 347-353, 354-360, 361-368, 377-386	191, 258-264, 265-272, 327-331	208-212	190, 273-281.			Balance 5.5:191 Machiavellianism 238-241

Investigator	Source	Field	9.1	1.9	1.1	5.5	9.9	Statistical 5.5	Facades	Paternalism	Other
Barber, J.D.	*The Presidential Character.* Englewood Cliffs, N.J.: Prentice-Hall. 1972.	Applied Politics Political Science	12-13,17-57,58-98, 99-142, 347-395, 413-442, 446-448	13,91, 173-206, 448-450	13,145-163,165, 166-167	170-173	12, 209-343, 452-454	79,86, 92-93	83	60,91	Two Hat: 86,87 Critique: 277-278, 331
Bell, G.D.	*The Achievers.* Chapel Hill, N.C.: Preston-Hill, Inc., 1973.	Business	23-38, 39-59, 132-152	73-83, 164-171	60-72, 153-163		104-124, 181-187		84-103, 172-180, 188-195		
Benne, K.D. & Sheats, P.	"Functional Roles of Group Members." *Journal of Social Issues* 4, no. 2 (1948): 41-49.	Clinical Psychology	45,46	44,45, 46	45	44	44		46		
Bennett, D.	*TA and the Manager.* New York: AMACON. 1976.	Business Consultant	14,19,26-27,30-32, 122,145 146-150, 161-162, 164-165, 230	14,26-27,32, 122,160-161,168-170,230-231	79,80, 145, 153,154, 160-161	18-19, 79-82, 129-137, 145,150-153	26-27, 81,82, 83,139-140,145, 154-157, 178,194-196,230		81,82, 91-116	231	Dom/Backup: 151-152, 181 Wide Arc: 230
Berne, E.	*Games People Play.* New York: Grove Press, 1964.	Psychiatry	27,112, 113	25-26			27, 178-179, 180-181, 182-183, 184		48-168		
Biestek, F.P.	*The Casework Relationship.* Chicago: Loyola U Press, 1957	Social Work	106-107	33-47	108	48-66	67-99, 100-119	23-32			
Bion, W.R.	*Experiences in Groups.* New York: Basic Books. 1959.	Psychoanalysis	152-153	147-150	152-153	150-152	156-158, 169				
Blake, R.R. & Mouton, J.S.	*The Grid for Sales Excellence: Benchmarks for Effective Salesmanship.* New York: McGraw-Hill. 1970.	Social Psychology	45-58	59-69	70-79	80-94	95-118	187	125-136	188	Dom/Backup: 13-15
Blake, R.R. & Mouton, J.S.	*The Grid for Supervisory Effectiveness.* Austin: Scientific Methods, Inc., 1975.	Social Psychology	11-28	29-43	44-58	59-78	79-107				Dom/Backup: 8-9

Investigator	Source	Field	9.1	1.9	1.1	5.5	9.9	Statistical 5.5	Facades	Paternalism	Other
Branden, N.	*The Psychology of Self-Esteem.* New York: Bantam Books, 1969.	Psychiatry	188-190	150,151	194-195	185-188	109-139, 146				
Burns, T. & Stalker, G.M.	*The Management of Innovation.* New York: Barnes & Noble, Social Science Paperbacks, 1961.	Organization Behavior	96-125				96-125				
Buzzotta, V.R., Lefton, R.E., Sherberg, M.	*Effective Selling Through Psychology: Dimensional Sales and Sales Management Strategies.* New York: Wiley Interscience, 1972.	Clinical Psychology	36-53, 99-100a, 120-121, 127,264-270,285-286,301-318,319, 320-324, 338-339, 344-347, 357-358, 358-359	68-82, 99-100a, 122,124, 127,274-277,287-288,301-318,319, 327-331, 340-341, 344-347, 358,359	54-67, 99-100a, 121,122, 127,270-274,286-287,301-318,319, 324,327, 339,340, 344-347, 358,359		83,98, 99-100a, 124,125, 127,199-224,277-283,288-289,301-318,319, 331-334, 341-343, 344-347, 358,359-360		113-117, 291-292		Dom/Backup: 101-112, 289-291
Durkheim, E.	"On Anomie." In C.W. Mills, ed. *Images of Man: The Classic Tradition in Sociological Thinking.* New York: George Braziller, Inc., 1960, pp. 449-485.	Sociology	455-461	460	460-461	449-461					

Investigator	Source	Field	9.1	1.9	1.1	5.5	9.9	Statistical 5.5	Facades	Paternalism	Other
Etzioni, A.	*A Comparative Analysis of Complex Organizations.* (Rev. ed.) New York: Free Press, 1975.	Sociology	xxiv,5-6, 8,12,15 27-31,56- 59,60-61, 66-67,75- 82,84,106 115,116- 118,133, 287,455- 460,471, 479,486- 490,500- 504		28,289	xxiv,5-6 6-8,12, 15,40-54, 56-59,61- 72,78,81- 82,89,92, 106,114- 117,169, 305-311, 426-427, 455-460, 471,479 486-490 500-504	471	433-436, 437-438		xxiv,5, 6-8,12, 15,31-39, 62-67,72- 75,78-82, 84-87,89, 106,112- 113,116, 271,389- 391,426- 427,455- 460,471, 479,486- 490,500- 504	Machiavel-lianism: 387
Fleishman, E.A.	"Twenty Years of Consideration and Structure." In E.A. Fleishman and J.G. Hunt, eds. *Current Developments in the Study of Leadership.* Carbondale: Southern Illinois University Press, 1973. pp. 1-40.	Industrial Psychology	25-26, 26-27, 29,32	23,25, 26-27, 29	26-27, 29,32, 36,37	29	23-24, 24-25, 26-27, 27-29, 32,35, 37	37			
Fromm, E.	*The Art of Loving.* London: Unwin Books, 1957.	Psychiatry	23,25, 31,43, 54-55	9,23,25, 42-43, 55-56	15-16, 23,83- 84	10-11, 18-22, 25,74- 76,80	24,26- 28,29, 42,53- 54,87, 104-109			82-83	
Gordon, T.	*Parent Effectiveness Training.* New York: Peter H. Wyden, 1970.	Counseling Psychology	10-11,41- 44,83-86, 110,112- 113,151, 152,153- 159,174- 183,195, 207,248, 260-261, 263,280, 321-322, 323-324, 325,326- 327	11,13-14, 43-44, 151,152, 154-155, 159-161, 184,190- 193,248, 251-253, 324-325, 326	44,152, 183,185, 327	42-43, 110,113, 184,289, 322,323, 324,325- 326,327,	12,30- 31,33, 47-61, 194-264, 280-282, 305-306	261-263	22-25	11,166, 168-169, 177-178, 190-191	Wide Arc: 11,161- 163

Investigator	Source	Field	9.1	1.9	1.1	5.5	9.9	Statistical 5.5	Facades	Paternalism	Other
Gordon, T.	*T.E.T.: Teacher Effectiveness Training.* New York: Peter H. Wyden, 1974.	Counseling Psychology	27-29,48-49,80-84,84-85,86-87,184-185,186-189,191,192-194,198-206,211-216	49,85-86,184,186-188,189-190,191,206-207	49,87,206-207,208-209	208	220-282			194-195,213	Dom/Backup: 23-24 Wide Arc: 190-191
Hardman, D.G.	*Authority Monograph.* National Council on Crime & Delinquency.	Social Work	219,245,246,248	215-217,219,249			249-255,245-254	217,221,247,249-255			
Harrington, A.	*The Immortalist.* Millbrae, Calif. Celestial Arts, 1977.	Philosophy	114,117,118,119,123-127,137,139		117,118,129-130	100-101,114-115,117,118,127-129	136-139		144-145	120-121	
Harris, T.A.	*I'm OK—You're OK.* New York: Avon, 1969.	Psychiatry	72-73,263	67-69	69-71,142-143,152	143-146,153	74-77,151-152,153,302-304		75-76,146-151,152,262-263		
Heath, R.	*The Reasonable Adventure:* Pittsburgh: The University of Pittsburgh Press, 1964.	Clinical Psychology	ix-x, xii 5-6,20-24,38,39,63-67	28-29		ix,xi,4-5,10-11,14-20,37-38,39,57-63	ix,x,7,8-10,30-36,39	x,xii-xiii,6-7,24-28,38,39,67-69			
Hersey, P. & Blanchard, K.H.	*Management and Organizational Behavior: Utilizing Human Resources.* (2nd ed.). Englewood Cliffs, N.J.: Prentice-Hall, 1972.	Education	35-37,46-48,61,63,70-76,92-93	61,63,74-76	70-76	74-76	46-48,61,63,70-76	83-86,121-123,127-131		61,63,133-143	Machiavellianism: 92-93 Wide Arc: 125 Change: 149-171

Investigator	Source	Field	9.1	1.9	1.1	5.5	9.9	Statistical 5.5	Facades	Paternalism	Other
Horney, K.	*Neurosis and Human Growth.* New York: W.W. Norton & Co., 1950.	Psychoanalysis	17-39,76, 97,191-213,214-215,304-306,311-316	76-77,97-98,215-238,239-243,316-324	43-44,77-78,259-290,304,324-328			312-315			Dom/Backup: 232-234 Sick 9.1: 247-256 Distorted 1.9:243-256
Horney, K.	*The Neurotic Personality of Our Time.* New York: W.W. Norton & Co., 1937.	Psychoanalysis	39,81-82, 98,162-187	36,85-87, 96-98, 102-161	99,191-192,212-213,237	28,96-97	104,107, 108,109, 113,163, 273-274	100-101			Distorted 1.9:259-280
Horney, K.	*Self-Analysis.* New York: W.W. Norton & Co., 1942.	Psychoanalysis	44,47-48, 56-57, 57-58, 58-59	54-55	48-52, 55-56, 57,58, 59-60, 62,108	58,108					Wide Arc: 44
James, M.	*The OK Boss.* Reading, Mass.: Addison-Wesley, 1975.	Adult Education	10-11,16-17,20-21, 35,36,39, 40,54,55, 56,57,59, 61,62,75, 76,77, 131,139,	13, 18-19,37, 39-40,75	14-15, 35,55, 56,57- 58,59- 61,62, 75-76, 135, 139-140	19,37, 77,132, 144	17,21, 54,55, 56,57, 59,61, 62,69, 76-77, 132-133, 139, 144-145, 161-163	27,38,64,	106-121, 124-127	12-13, 35,36, 39,73-75	Dom/Backup: 8-9
James, M. & Jongeward, D.	*Born To Win: Transactional Analysis with Gestalt Experiments.* Reading, Mass.: Addison-Wesley, 1971.	Education	18,36,68-100,101-126,230	18,37, 127-159, 230-231	37,50, 56-57	18,57-58, 58-59, 224-226	18,36, 56,62, 235-238, 263-274	2-3, 227-228	29-35, 58	86, 229-230	
Jennings, E.E.	*The Executive Autocrat, Bureaucrat, Democrat.* New York: Harper & Row, 1962.	Business Education	2,4,20-21,25,66-70,75-77, 83-86,86-90,114-163			2,4,90-91,91-97, 105-106, 164-195, 228-232	2-3,4, 59-61, 97-106, 196-234	77-80, 256-266	85,250	25-26, 149, 157-160	Dom/Backup: 117
Jung, C.G.	*Psychological Types.* Princeton: Princeton University Press, 1971.	Psychiatry	346-354, 383-387		385-386, 388-391, 395-398, 401-403, 403-405	334-335, 354-355, 356-359, 363-366		368-370	384		Dom/Backup: 355-356, 362-363, 405-407

Investigator	Source	Field	9.1	1.9	1.1	5.5	9.9	Statistical 5.5	Facades	Paternalism	Other
Kangas, J.A. & Solomon, G.H.	*The Psychology of Strength.* Englewood Cliffs, N.J.: Prentice-Hall. 1975.	Psychology	7-9,10-11, 14,15-17, 55-56, 56-57, 135-136	18-19,22, 24,78	20-21, 21-22, 23	11-12, 19, 57-58	3,9,12, 21,23- 24,24- 25,68- 69,117, 130-135, 136-141, 142-145, 146-150, 151-168	26-27	13-14,17- 18,19-20, 24-25,29- 30,56,77		Wide Arc: 136
Kovar, L.C.	*Faces of the Adolescent Girl.* Englewood Cliffs, N.J.: Prentice-Hall. 1968.	Adolescent Psychology	11-12, 73-83, 103-106	9-10, 53-68	79	10-11, 35-51, 83, 148-149	4-9, 107-125, 148-149				
Kunkel, F.M. & Dickerson, R.E.	*How Character Develops: A Psychological Interpretation.* New York: Charles Scribner & Sons. 1946.	Psychology	68-81	60-67	80-82		125-140, 157-159, 176-178				
Leary, T.	*Interpersonal Diagnosis of Personality.* New York: Ronald Press. 1957.	Clinical Psychology	19,64-65, 104,105, 135,137, 233,269- 281,324- 331,332- 340	64-65, 104,105, 135,233, 292-302, 303-314	19,23-24, 64-65,95- 96,104, 105,135, 233,282- 291	19,64-65, 135,202- 203,233, 315-322	21,64-65, 135,233, 323-324		181-186, 188-191, 282-283, 284-285, 316,317, 318,324, 325,326	64-65, 93	Dom/Backup: 225-227 Distorted 1.9:284- 286,288- 289,367 Sick 9.1: 341-350, 354,372
Likert, R.	*The Human Organization: Its Management and Value.* New York: McGraw-Hill. 1967.	Organization Behavior	3-12, 13-46			3-12, 13-46	3-12, 13-46, 47-100			3-12, 13-46	

Investigator	Source	Field	9.1	1.9	1.1	5.5	9.9	Statistical 5.5	Facades	Paternalism	Other
Likert, R. & Likert, J.G.	New Ways of Managing Conflict. New York: McGraw-Hill, 1976.	Organization Behavior	19-40, 59-69			19-40	16-17, 19-40, 49-51, 51-56, 71-324			19-40	
McClelland, D.C.	Power: The Inner Experience. New York: Irvington Publishers, 1975.	Individual Psychology	7-8, 8-12, 13-21, 27, 49-51, 52-76, 77-78, 249, 252-254, 255-256, 257, 258, 260-261, 264, 266, 274-275, 295-297-324, 326, 328	27, 104-122, 255, 264, 274, 289, 322-323, 325, 328		27, 155, 157-158, 249	27, 257, 258-260, 261, 261-263, 263, 266, 269, 288, 301-302, 324, 325, 329		301-302	35-36, 142-144, 260, 289-290	Distorted 1.9:102, 104 Sick 9.1: 255 OD:254, 255
McGregor, D.	The Human Side of Enterprise. New York: McGraw-Hill, 1960.	Psychology	33-43				45-57, 61-246				
McGregor, D.	The Professional Manager. New York: McGraw-Hill, 1967.	Psychology	59-63, 79-80, 117-118, 118-125, 136-137, 138-140, 148-149	59-63	59-63	59-63, 144-145	29-30, 59-63, 79-80, 118-127-130, 130-133, 140, 162-182, 191-195			7-10, 142-144	Dom/Backup: 60
Maccoby, M.	The Gamesman. New York: Simon & Schuster, 1976.	Psychiatry	34, 47-48, 76-85, 181-182, 183-184, 187-189, 212-213	183-187	94	34, 35, 46-47, 48, 50-75, 86-97, 189-209	179, 212, 213-217	100, 149	48-49, 91, 92-93, 98-120, 121-171	240-241	

Investigator	Source	Field	9,1	1,9	1,1	5,5	9,9	Statistical 5,5	Facades	Pater-nalism	Other
May, R.	*Love and Will.* New York: W. W. Norton & Co., 1969.	Clinical Psychology	45-48, 57-59, 276-278	278-279	27-33	40-45, 279	55-56, 91-92, 146.283-286.303-304.306, 310-311				
Meininger. J.	*Success Through Transactional Analysis.* New York: New American Library, 1973.	Business Consultant	26-27, 28-29, 33.39-40.43-44.64-67.73-75.87-90,128-129	29-30, 34-36, 38.43-44.45-46.67-71.75-76.90-92,105-106,166-170,186-190	36.39-40.40-42.43-44.56-57,100-101,105-106,110-113,153,157	30-31, 57-60, 76-77	26-27, 36.37, 63-64, 101,113-114,129-130,158-160,165-166,175-177,178-185,186-206	66	7-10.60-63.78-99. 106-109. 173-175	153, 160-161	Wide Arc: 66 Change: 132-139, 194-204
Metcalf, H.C. & Urwick, L.	*Dynamic Administration: The Collected Papers of Mary Parker Follett:* New York: Harper & Bros., 1940.	Government and Administration	31.50-58. 96-101, 272-277	190		31-32.35, 210-213, 239	31. 33-49, 58-70, 111-116, 198-202		213-225, 240-246, 260-269. 279-281		
Missildine, W.H.	*Your Inner Child of the Past.* New York: Simon & Schuster, 1963.	Psychiatry	77.85-100,103, 106,108-109,125-126-130-133,138-139	77,133-136,157, 166,171-191,259-260,266-267,271-272	78-79. 101-103, 104-105, 107-108, 109-111, 121-124, 145-155, 156-159, 165-166, 166-167, 243-252, 254-259, 261						

Investigator	Source	Field	9.1	1.9	1.1	5.5	9.9	Statistical 5.5	Facades	Paternalism	Other
Missildine, W.H. & Galton, L.	*Your Inner Conflicts— How to Solve Them.* New York: Simon & Schuster, 1974.	Psychiatry	35-36,37, 38-39,39- 40,62,72- 74,76,77, 81-82, 83-86, 131-133, 145-146, 154-155, 171-172, 172-180, 187-191, 196-201, 205-207	36,37- 38,61, 76-77, 130	37,39, 53-59, 60-60- 61,62, 62-63, 77, 120-127, 157-160, 162-163, 184-187		33-34, 262-263, 308-313				
Moment, D. & Zaleznik, A.	*Role Development and Interpersonal Competence.* Boston: Harvard University Press, 1963.	Business Administration	20,38,56, 62-63,67, 72,77,80, 85-86,87- 88,89, 104-105, 122-123, 158-159, 160	20,39, 56,62- 63,67, 72,77, 78-79, 80,83, 86-87, 89, 105-106, 123-124, 159-160	20,36- 37,39, 56,62- 63,67, 72,80, 83,87, 89-90, 106-107, 124-125		19-20, 36-37, 38,41, 53,56, 62-63, 68,72, 77,80, 85,89, 104, 120-122				
Mouton, J.S. & Blake, R.R.	*The Marriage Grid* New York: McGraw-Hill, 1971.	Social Psychology	41-67	97-113	123-137	151-169	181-201	80-85	76-80	69-74	Dom/Backup: 15-17
Reddin, W.J.	*Managerial Effectiveness 3-D.* New York: McGraw-Hill, 1970.	Business Administration	27,28-29, 31-32,42, 47,73-74, 94-95, 161,177, 192,194, 194-195, 221-227, 262,263, 268-269	27,28-29, 31,42,68, 73,94, 194,215- 219	43,48, 54,194, 209-212, 258-259, 263,264.	27,28-29, 30-31,41, 42-43,48, 72-73, 93-94, 194,205- 209,213, 231-233	27,28- 29,32, 41,48, 74-75, 94,95, 192,194, 230-231, 233-234	52,53-54, 139-140, 149-150, 159-160, 169-178, 181-185, 256-257		42,47	Dom/Backup: 46-47,48, 49,152 Change: 163,307
Reid, W. & Epstein, L.	*Task-Centered Casework.* New York: Columbia U Press, 1972.	Social Work		155-156		136-138	1-260				

Investigator	Source	Field	9.1	1.9	1.1	5.5	9.9	Statistical 5.5	Facades	Paternalism	Other
Riesman, D., Glazer, N., & Denney, R.	*The Lonely Crowd* Garden City, N.Y.: Doubleday & Co., 1953.	Sociology Political Science Economic History	23,28-32, 41,57-63		278,281	23,24-28, 33,34-40, 41-42, 63-74, 278	33,278, 282,286-298,328		302-305, 305-307	303	
Roberts, R.W. & Nee, R.H.	*Theories of Social Casework.* Chicago: U of Chicago Press, 1970	Social Work	181-218	33-75, 131-179			77-128, 313-351				
Schutz, W.C.	*The Interpersonal Underworld* (originally titled *FIRO: A Three Dimensional Theory of Interpersonal Behavior).* Palo Alto, Calif.: Science & Behavior Books, 1966.	Psychology	29,41,46, 47-48,89	31,36,41, 47,48,89	25-26, 28-29, 30-31, 41,42, 45-46, 47,48, 89	26-27	27,29-30,31, 37,41, 43,48, 87-89			43	Sick 9,1: 43 Distorted 1,9:42-43
Steiner, C.M.	*Scripts People Live: Transactional Analysis of Life Scripts.* New York: Bantam Books, 1974.	Therapy	53,54-46, 78-81, 115-119, 188-193, 197-198, 231-234, 236-237, 253-261	54,56, 76-78, 198-201, 211-213, 222-224	92-95, 115-119, 178-181, 218-220, 243-245		3,85-86, 352-361, 362-370, 382-383, 384		44-50, 121, 175-178, 304-305		Wide Arc: 39 Dom/Backup: 37-38

Investigator	Source	Field	9.1	1.9	1.1	5.5	9.9	Statistical 5.5	Facades	Paternalism	Other
Thomas, W.I. & Znaniecki, F.	"Three Types of Personality." In C.W. Mills, ed., *Images of Man: The Classic Tradition in Sociological Thinking.* New York: George Braziller, Inc., 1960, pp. 405-436.	Sociology	427			407-408, 409,411, 418-419, 421,423, 425,427, 428,434, 435-436	408,409, 411,418, 423,435, 436	408-409, 418,423, 433,435, 436		420	
Wheelis, A.	*The Quest for Identity.* New York: W.W. Norton & Co., 1958.	Psychiatry	18,85			18-19, 48-49, 85-89, 91-93, 126	19,20	85			
White, R. & Lippitt, R.	"Leader Behavior and Member Reaction in Three 'Social Climates.'" In D. Cartwright and A. Zander, eds., *Group Dynamics: Research and Theory.* (2nd ed.) Evanston, Ill.: Row, Peterson, & Co., 1960, pp. 527-553.	Social Psychology	528-529, 529-532, 537,540-541,541-546,549-553		528-529, 530,531, 533-534, 539-540, 549-552	528-529, 530,531, 532-538, 539-541, 546-549, 549-553					

INDEX

155